Feed Your Brain

A Guide to Eating for Optimal Mental Health

Tonya Monique Peavy, PsyD

And

Le'Andra Scott, B.A.

This book is dedicated to all the beautiful people in world who desire to live in overall good health—mind, body, and spirit.

Feed Your Brain: A Guide to Eating for Optimal Mental Health

First published in February 2019

Copyright © 2019 Dr. Tonya M. Peavy, Psy.D. and Le'Andra R. Scott

This book or parts thereof may not be reproduced in any form, stored in a retrieval system or transmitted in any form by any means—electronic, mechanical, photocopy, recording, or otherwise—without prior written permission of the publisher, or the authors.

ISBN: 978-1726209762

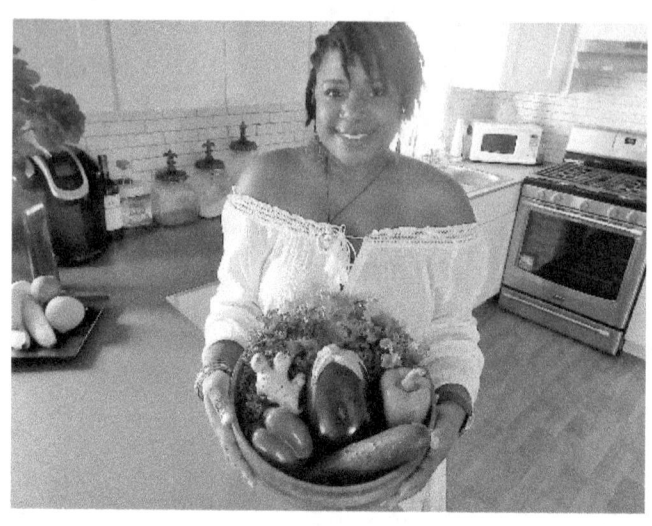

Dr. Tonya Peavy, Psy.D.

Dr. Tonya Peavy is an emotional healing practitioner, licensed professional counselor, adjunct psychology professor, Master Reiki Practitioner, and TESOL certified English teacher. She holds a doctorate in clinical psychology, master's degree in counseling psychology, and bachelor's degree in child and family development. She is a mental health expert and holistic nutrition enthusiast whose mission through her teachings is to educate and inspire optimal mental wellness. Dr. Tonya's work focuses on revitalization of mental wellness. She also maintains a tele-health practice. Her interests are practicing yoga, holistic nutrition, body movement healing, and loving all life forms. She currently resides in South America.

Website/Blog: www.drpeavypsyd.com

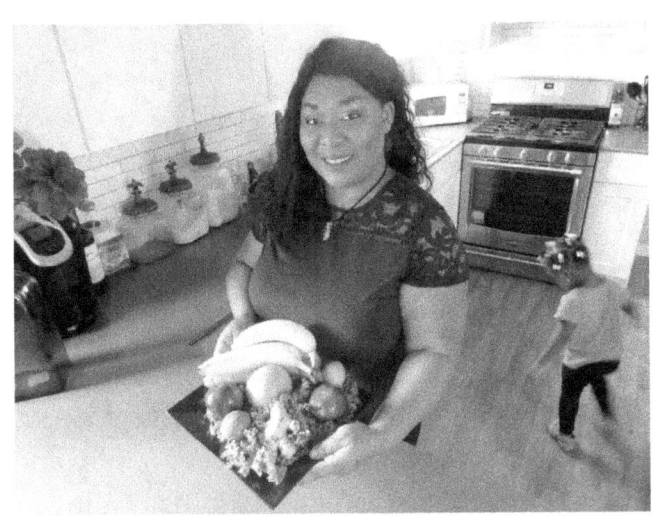

Le'Andra Scott, B.A.

Le'Andra Scott is an administrative healthcare professional, visual artist and food enthusiast. She holds a bachelor's degree in art and has completed coursework towards a master's degree in clinical Mental Health Counseling. With her love for food, she takes an untraditional approach in preparing meals for her family. Her inspiration comes from her research in herbs from renowned resources such as Dr. Afrika and the late-Dr. Sebi. Le'Andra Scott has found that herbs not only provide great health benefits but can also make foods flavorful. She is currently preparing to enter certification program in herbal medicine and nutrition.

Website/Blog: www.purplestargoddess.com
IG: @purplestargoddess
YouTube: Purple Star Goddess

Note to the Reader

This book was written with the expertise of, co-author Dr. Tonya Peavy, a mental health professional who treat individuals in inpatient and outpatient settings. In those experiences, it was noted that most individuals maintained poor dietary habits and those who did not, simply were not aware of foods and herbs that could improve their mental well-being. Co-author LeAndra Scott has self-studied herbal remedies from renowned sources for five years and has archived remedies that worked for herself, family and friends. Both authors partnered to further study the healing benefits of foods and herbs and collaborated to develop a guide for that could be used to help others.

This book is to be used as tool guide to enhance your dietary awareness for better mental health. The information, tips, and suggestions should not replace the advice of your physician. Please discuss with your physician and/or pharmacist about interactions that may occur with your prescribed medications.

Be enlightened. Be healthy. Be happy.

~ Dr. Tonya and Le'Andra

Optimal Use of the Guide

Chapter Two, by far, is the richest source of information as it details the function of neurotransmitters and the nutrients that stimulate them, as well as the foods that contain such nutrients. After you have read Chapter Two, you will have a better understanding of the bases of how nutrients from food contributes to our overall mental well-being.

We have broken the book into chapters by common ailments. In the subsequent chapters, you will learn more about the ailments but, importantly, under the "Optimal Nutritional Suggestions" section, you will find the specific food and recipes to improve your mental well-being for that ailment.

Table of Contents

Authors.. 4-5

Note to Reader...6

Optimal Use of Guide.................................... 7

Introduction... 10

Chapter 1: Mental Health............................12

Chapter 2: Nutrition & Mental Health.............19

Chapter 3: Depression................................. 39

Chapter 4: Stress & Anxiety..........................49

Chapter 5: Attention-Deficit & Hyperactivity... 63

Chapter 6: Cognitive Decline........................ 72

Chapter 7: Psychosis...................................82

References... 92

The TEA!..96

Journal Page...99

Mental Resources..100

Introduction

Mental health is an important part of your physical health and own well-being. When there is suffering and a diminished functioning in your day-to-day as it relates to your physical health, you refer to it as illness. Well, the same is true for your mental health. There are illnesses that are temporary (acute) and those that require management throughout your lifespan (chronic); this is true for physical and mental illness. Whether identified as a disorder or just symptoms, illness makes us feel unwell, and unprepared for ordinary daily activities.

Everyone, at least once, in their lifetime will experience, illness of the psyche at any degree. In fact, nearly 20% of American adults will experience mental illness in any year. Just as we adopt hygiene habits for physical care, it is equally important to incorporate good mental hygiene practices for prevention or management of mental health disorders. There are traditional forms of treating mental illness through a combination of medication and/or psychotherapy. However, food planning as a mean of treatment is seldom discussed when it comes to mental illness. We attribute "bad food" to physical health and not how it affects are brains. For optimal health, the brain requires various essential fatty acids, complex carbohydrates, amino acids, vitamins and minerals, and water.

Chapter 1

Mental Health

"Your mental health is a priority. Your happiness is an essential. Your self-care is a necessity."
~ HealthyPlace.Com

Overview of Mental Health

According to the World Health Organization (2014), mental health is a state well-being in which a person acknowledges their own abilities, can manage daily stresses of life, can work efficiently, and is able to be a productive participant in their community. In fact, there are numerous ways to define mental health. Such as above, most definitions emphasize positive psychological well-being. Alternatively, others may define mental health as the absence of mental health problems.

In this book, mental health is viewed on a continuum of having good mental hygiene to having a mental disorder. It is important to understand that a person may vary on this continuum at any point in their lives. A person demonstrating good mental hygiene is someone who can regulate their emotions, maintain positive relationships with others, and have sound cognitive functioning. Good mental hygiene means that a person actively practices the prevention or management of mental health disorders. When practices are good standards of mental health, it allows a person to demonstrate optimal performance at in multiple facets of their lives, including home, work, and in social settings. It must be noted that at any time in life you may experience breakdown in mental wellness.

Defining Mental Health

There are a variety of terms that are used interchangeably to describe mental health concerns, such as mental illness, mental disorder, emotional disturbance, psychiatric illness, nervous breakdown, mental exhaustion, or burnout. There are more unfavorable terms used, that can be associated with mental health stigma, such as wacky, psycho, crazy, not wrapped too tight, nuts, insane, or loony. These common descriptors poorly provide information about the person's experience.

When a person experiences physical pain that interrupts their overall well-being; he or she will seek medical attention or find the best over-the-counter remedy to feel well. The terms psychiatric illness or mental illness are most appropriate to understanding what the person is experiencing when they are feeling emotionally, or cognitively unwell. A **mental disorder** is a diagnosable illness that affects all areas of functioning in a person's life— emotions, thinking, and behavior, and disruption to a person's ability to work, perform activities of daily living, and maintain personal relationships. With a physical illness, whether a person has received a diagnosis by a medical professional or not, it does not lessen the fact of feeling unwell. The same is true for mental illness, a person may not have gone to a professional for treatment, but he or she are still vulnerable to illness the same. Mental illness are thought to be the result of a combination of factors, including age, biological and environmental factors.

Mental Health Disorders in the United States

The Diagnostic and Statistical Manual of Mental Disorders, fifth edition (DSM-5) is used to diagnose mental disorders. There are different types of mental illnesses, but for this book, we are going to explore some of the common mental disorders or symptoms that can be managed with nutrition. Common disorders or symptoms that I treat in private practice and psychiatric outpatient programs are depression, anxiety, mood disorders (bipolar disorder), attention deficit-hyperactivity disorder (ADHD), poor memory, psychosis, and autism.

In the United States, mental disorders are common and are found one in five adults in any year (CBHSQ, 2015). Research found that nearly 19 percent of adults (18 or older) experienced a mental illness in any one year, which is equivalent to almost 44 million people. This study, conducted in 2014, reflects the entire population of the United States and may indicate higher or lower rates in mental disorders in subgroups. This is mainly because some mental health disorders are co-morbid. Other terms for describing a simultaneous combination of mental disorders are dual diagnosis, or co-occurrence. Let's take a look at what this really means. As a mental health practitioner, Dr. Peavy treat individuals with various diagnoses. Many of the individuals treated for depression are likely to be treated for anxiety as well. Likewise, the individuals that treated for mood disorders and/or psychosis are likely to need treatment for substance abuse. Of the U.S. adults with mental disorders, nearly 14% have at least one disorder, almost 6% have two disorders, and more than 6% have three or more disorders.

TABLE 1. Mental Disorder Percentages

MENTAL DISORDER	ADULTS
Anxiety Disorders	18%
Major Depressive Disorder	7%
Mood Disorders (Bipolar Disorders)	3%
Psychotic Disorders	1%
Other Mental Disorders (including ADHD, Autism)	18.5%

Significance of Mental Disorders

If you are tuned into pop culture or social media, there are hashtags, slogans, and all types of public service announcements (PSA) attempting to bring awareness to mental illness and its impact in our community (e.g. #OkayToSay, #BreakingTheSilence, #BreakingTheStigma, #CureStigma, #mentalillnesslookslike). These national campaigns are in response to many years of marginalization of individuals attempting to navigate mental health problems that lead to mass incarcerations, academic problems, unemployment, discrimination, and even, suicide. Mental disorders are disabilities that are not as visible to others, and this poses a risk if the public is not aware because these individuals are likely be judged as lazy, stubborn, or not ill which lead to individuals isolating themselves.

Research as shown that nearly fifty percent of all mental health disorders began by age 14 and seventy-five percent are developed before age 25 (Kessler et. al, 2005). During my work as assistant director of admissions in a psychiatric hospital, often time these statistics were representative of the individuals that I evaluated for treatment—they were many times younger than age 14. The youngest individual that I evaluated for psychiatric admission was age 3. When mental illness begins at an early age, it affects youth's academic achievement, maturation into the adult workforce, formation of social relationships, and risk of substance use. Subsequently, mental illness can lead to disability throughout a person's life. It is most important to identify problems early to ensure the person receives proper treatment and care.

Current Approach to Mental Health Treatment

There are various treatment modalities used to treat and provide support for mental illness. The type of treatment recommended will vary by mental health complaint or symptoms. Remember, there is no "one size fits all" approach. The best course treatment should be planned by a professional which includes, a licensed mental health professional (e.g. psychologist, professional counselor, clinical social worker, marriage and family counselor or psychiatric nurse) or psychiatrist. How do you know when a licensed mental health professional versus a psychiatrist is needed? Here's a quick breakdown:

- **Psychiatrists** are medical doctors who specialize in the treatment of mental disorders that are severe and/or long-lasting disorders which require medication to effectively management the disorder (e.g. psychotic disorders, severe major depression, bipolar disorders, panic disorder, etc.).

- **Licensed mental health professionals** (i.e. psychologists, licensed counselors, clinical social workers, and psychiatric nurses) are master or doctoral-degreed professionals who specialize in the treatment of mental health issues. Although, they are not medical doctors, some states allow psychologists and nurse practitioners to prescribe medications used to treat mental health issues.

- **Primary Care Physicians** are medical doctors who are, likely to be, the first health professionals a person seek when experiencing psychological distress. They are trained to recognize developing symptoms and make referrals to trained mental health professionals as needed. They sometimes prescribe medications to manage psychological distress, but do not offer therapeutic interventions.

The following are treatment methods used by mental health professionals:

- **Medication Management**, or psychopharmacology is treatment using medications prescribed by physician, a prescribing psychologist, or psychiatric nurse.

- **Psychotherapy, Therapy,** or **Counseling** is treatment involving talking with a professional to help explore past experiences, change harmful thought patterns, and/or ways of behaving that are distressing for the person or people around them.

For decades the most prevalent treatments for mental health problems has been medication and psychotherapy. One of the clearest, yet unheralded factors in the development of major trends in mental health is the role of nutrition.

Chapter 2

Nutrition and Mental Health

"Let food be thy medicine and medicine be thy food".
~Hippocrates

The Link between Physical and Mental Health

For some individuals, alternative modalities of therapy bind collectively with traditional methods of treating mental health problems. For example, a person prescribed medication for depression, may find additional benefits from adding certain foods or herbs to their diet to increase mood. As practitioners continue a path of using medication and psychotherapy, one area that is receiving increasing attention from several communities is the role of nutrition in mental health. Nutrition has a serious stake in this match as a possible alternative or supplemental treatment in the emerging integrative approach to treating individuals. In the past ten years, there has been a growing number of publications describing and validating alternative approaches in mental health. Both anecdotal and clinical evidence have supported the links between physical activity, spirituality, acupuncture, and diet.

For the past decade, the United States has been in battle to save individuals from obesity and obesity related illnesses. Therefore, most individuals in the U.S. are aware of the well-documented association between diet and physical health.

For instance, we know there are strong implications in the development of coronary heart disease (CHD), Type 2 diabetes, and some cancers, if we maintain a diet in high in saturated fats, salt, and sugar and low in fruit, vegetables, and fiber.

In the United States, it is less common to discuss the similar association between nutrition and mental health. Indeed, the contribution of nutrition to our mental health is intricate and wholeheartedly affected by other issues, there is an unassuming belief acknowledged by those who embrace an integrative wellness—nutrition affects physical health and physical health affects the mind. In other words, what we eat contributes to how we feel and behave.

FIGURE 1. The Integrated Association between Diet, Physical Health, and Mental Health

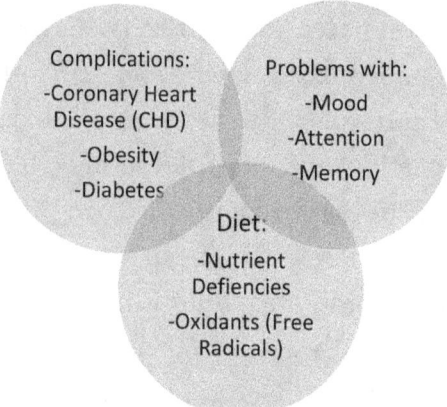

Understanding the Well-Fed Brain

Co-author of this book, Dr. Peavy was not always attuned to feeding the brain. So, let us share her story with you. Dr.

Peavy was beaming with excitement when she moved to Brooklyn, New York; she could hardly sleep and could not get enough of street food. Well...eventually, she had enough. She had become violently ill after consuming an improperly cooked and/or stored lamb gyro. As expected, her stomach recoiled, but, for some reason, later she did not associate her increased poor concentration, memory fogginess, and irritability to food. For many of us, we have experienced the," Was it something that I ate?" moment when it comes to physical symptoms. However, we likely do not apply this instinct to food affecting the brain — our mental health.

Perhaps the health of our brain is seldom a significant factor in our dietary concerns because the brain has a quality of complexity unlike other vital organs. It does not cause immediate pain in the way that our stomachs might wince after an incident of food poisoning, so it is less likely for us to learn to associate what we eat to how our brain responds. Nevertheless, like other vital organs, the brain is highly sensitive to our daily dietary intake. For optimal health, the brain requires various amounts of the following vital nutrients:

1. Essential Fatty Acids
2. Complex Carbohydrates
3. Amino Acids
4. Vitamins and Minerals
5. Water

By now, we know you are ready to get to the nitty gritty of what to eat! Please bear with us because before you can fully understand the impact of nutrients in the brain, we thought it would be helpful to understand the brain's communication process.

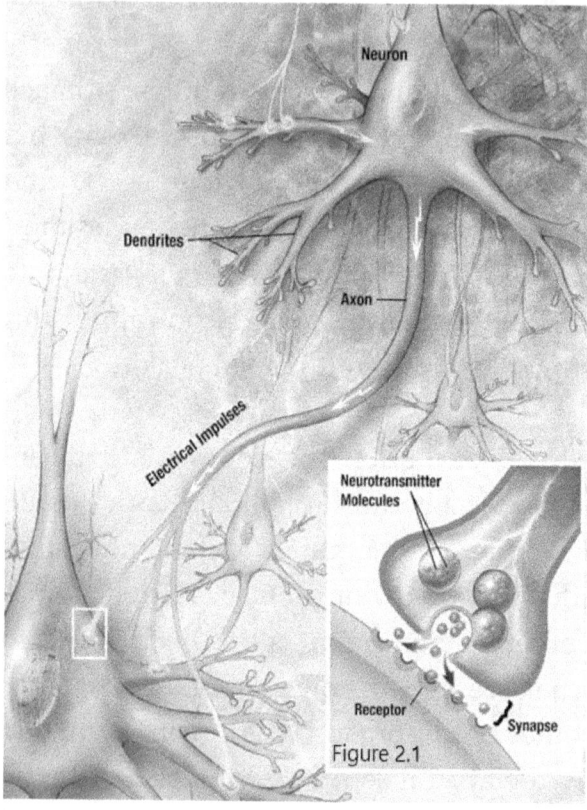

FIGURE 2. Communication in the Brain

The brain is somewhat composed of billions of nerve cells, known as **neurons**. Neurons allow the brain to communicate within itself and throughout the rest of the nervous system. Each neuron is connected to thousands of other neurons by branches called **axons** and **dendrites**. Each neuron, axon and dendrite are chiefly composed of unsaturated fat (lipids) that allows them to move quickly and these are derived from the diet. Between each branch, **neurotransmitters** (a gap, shown in Figure 2.1) pass messages back and forth. These messages allow neurons to communicate information amongst themselves. Neurotransmitters are made from amino acids, which often must be derived directly from the diet. Keep this in mind because it is about to become clearer!

Understanding the Foods that Deceive and Harm the Brain

There are four neurotransmitters that are important when it comes to our thoughts and general mood:

- acetylcholine
- serotonin
- dopamine including adrenaline/noradrenaline
- 4-aminobutyrate (GABA)

An adequate balance of these neurotransmitters is vital for good mental health because they are influential in feelings of pleasure, anxiety, memory and reasoning. When an individual has a neurotransmitter imbalance or deficiency, it manifests a host of symptoms that range from lack of motivation to sleep disturbances, or anxiety. You will learn more about how food impacts neurotransmitters later in the chapter.

How Food Can Deceive the Brain

There are substances that are divine at temporarily stimulating the neurotransmitter that is imbalanced or deficient. Have you ever experienced a strong craving and after consuming the food and that euphoric feeling followed afterwards? Well, as we eat foods that (our mind) are craving, they perform a magic trick of making us feel better for a while. For example, if an individual is low in levels of acetylcholine, they may find themselves craving junk foods, sugar, or fried foods; when these foods are consumed, they give short-term boost to levels of acetylcholine (which is responsible for memory and organized thoughts).

Likewise, when there are low levels of dopamine, a person may feel a lack of motivation or depressed, however, eating chocolate can boost feelings of enthusiasm and happiness. Individuals who use nicotine products may complain of "feeling on edge" without it, but report feeling relaxed after use; this is due to the release of dopamine and GABA. Although, we may have all experienced the immediate psychological effects of at least one of these products, the process is of trickery, or deception over the long term. When the long-standing process of this trickery exists, the brain becomes less sensitive to its own transmitters and has difficulty being able to produce healthy patterns of brain activity.

We're sure the next mood-altering culprit sounds familiar. Have you ever rewarded your child with a tasty treat? Yes, we're speaking of a sweet treat. This delight might bring about a little song and/or dance because.... you're the best! If that treat contains large amounts of sugar, you may notice a change in the child's mood and behavior. Most times, when children have consumed too much sugar, their activity level increases and their ability to focus decreases. Yikes! This is believed to be attributed to how sugar excites several neurotransmitters — (increased) dopamine, (increased) acetylcholine, and (decreased) GABA from the pancreas.

Natural sap from sugar cane, or raw sugar cane juice is rich in antioxidant phenols, however those antioxidants are destroyed by the heat in the process of making refined sugar — the sugar commonly used in most processed foods. This sugar excites a surge in dopamine — the reward system of our brain where we get that feeling of pleasure. In other words, sugar can produce a similar effect to doing a drug like heroin which brings a flood of dopamine. Likewise, refined sugar as an effect on acetylcholine production. Acetylcholine is found in the brain and in neurons in the muscles; it plays a role in arousal, attention, and motor function. Glucose (sugar) in a meal naturally increases the production of acetylcholine which increases at the end of a meal. If sugar is consumed in excessive amounts, it stimulates muscle energy and brain function. Thus, this appears as hyperactivity and inattentiveness due to the over stimulation in brain activity. 4-Aminobutyrate, or GABA, is the regulator among the neurotransmitters; it works to reduce excitability—keeping the effects of dopamine in balance. In the pancreas, GABA is produced as a result of glucose stimulation in the B cells (where insulin is produced). When sugar is consumed in excessive amounts, production of GABA is decreased causing an increase in excitability—hyperactivity.

How Food Can Harm the Brain

Just as we have foods that deceive the brain by releasing or suppressing vital neurotransmitters, there are foods that harm the brain with the release of oxidants, or free radicals that are toxic in the body. Oxidants are unstable molecules, missing electrons, which hate the feeling of being out of balance. Consequently, they steal what they need from other cells, creating more damaged, unbalanced free radicals that in turn steal electrons from other healthy cells. Needless to say, it is a brutal cycle that wreak havoc. Though normal cell functions produce a small percentage of oxidants, some foods can increase their emission to a level that the places strain on the body.

Saturated fats (e.g. whole milk products, butter, and lard) and trans-fats (hydrogenated, refined and hardened unsaturated vegetable oils) are two of the worst offenders in this category. Oxidants have been linked to certain cancers, heart disease, and other age-related diseases. The benefit of adding lean protein, fresh fruits and vegetables (which are high antioxidants), and herbs in recipes can maximize your overall health. In the next section, we will explore effective ways to increase the body's natural ability to fight toxins and explore foods that will provide nourishment to the brain. Table 2 summarizes the effects of deficiency in each of neurotransmitters, the foods that will make the deficiency worse and those that will improve it.

Table 2. Summary of Neurotransmitter Deficiency and Foods

Neurotransmitter	Deficiency Effects	Avoid	Consume
Acetylcholine	-Disorganization -Memory Loss -Loss of Creativity	Sugar, Fast Food (Fried), Processed Foods, Alcohol	Eggs, Wild Caught Fish (Mackerel, Salmon, Sardines, Tuna
Dopamine (adrenaline/noradrenaline)	-Stimulant Cravings -Low Motivation -Low Interest -Inattentiveness	Caffeinated (i.e. black tea, coffee, soft drinks, diet pills)	Balanced Diet with Vitamin C rich Fruit & Vegetables, Wheat germ, Green Tea
Serotonin	-Low Mood -Sleep Disturbance -Uneasiness -Impulsivity	Alcohol	Avocado, Eggs, Cheese, Fruit (Pineapple), Fish Turkey
GABA	-Irritability -Anxious Thoughts -Feeling Keyed Up -Self-deprecating	Sugar, Alcohol, Caffeinated Beverages	Bananas, Eggs Dark Green Veggies, Nuts Seeds

Understanding Foods and Nutrients that Feed the Brain

As mentioned earlier, we learned that some nutrients deceive the brain by activating an excessive release of neurotransmitters and some foods harm the brain by releasing oxidants, or toxins that damage healthy brain cells. Both processes are associated in acute (short-term) and chronic (long-term) mental health issues. Luckily, there are several nutrients that help the brain without deception or harm and can increase mood and mental wellness. These nutrients are known to contain antioxidants because they remove potentially damaging oxidizing agents (see Figure 3). In this section, we will explore the role of essential fatty acids, complex carbohydrates, amino acids, vitamin and minerals, and water.

Figure 3. Antioxidants Neutralizing Oxidants (Free Radicals)

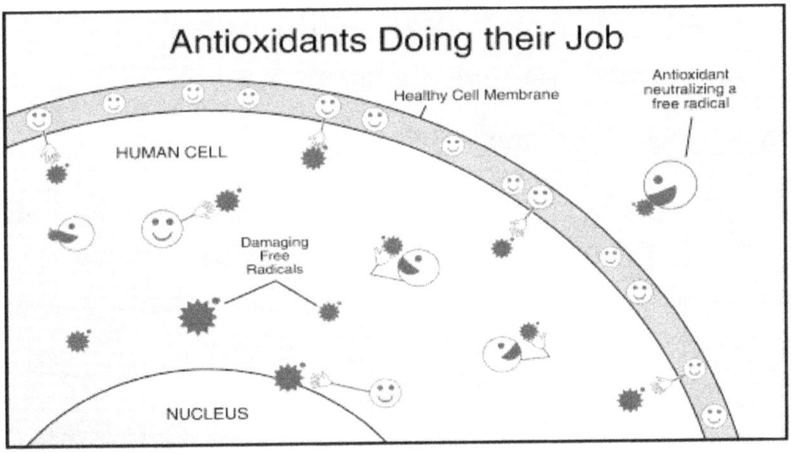

Antioxidants Doing their Job

Essential Fatty Acids

All fats, including saturated fatty acids, have important roles in the body. However, the most important fats are those that the body cannot produce and thus must come from the food we eat. These essential fatty acids (EFAs) are based on linoleic acid (omega-6 group) and alpha-linolenic acid (omega-3 group). Both groups of essential fatty acids are paramount to our survival. A deficiency in EFAs have been linked to attention deficits, depression, schizophrenia, and neurological disorders like Alzheimer's disease and Parkinson's.

Optimal Choices for Omega-3 EFAs (Linolenic Acid)

- Cold water high-fat fish, wild Alaskan salmon, sardines, anchovies, mackerel, shad, herring, and trout
- Flaxseed oil (the highest linolenic content of any food), flaxseeds, flaxseed meal, hempseed oil, hempseeds, walnuts, pumpkin seeds, brazil nuts, and sesame seeds
- Avocados
- Certain dark green leafy vegetables such as kale, spinach, purslane, mustard greens, and collards

Optimal Choices for Omega-6 EFAs (Linoleic Acid)

- Flaxseed oil, hempseed oil, grapeseed oil, borage oil, evening primrose oil, black currant seed (black seed) oil
- Flaxseeds, flaxseed meal, hemp seeds, pumpkin seeds and raw sunflower seeds
- Nuts, including pine nuts and pistachios
- Acai

Complex Carbohydrates

Complex carbohydrates, or "complex carbs" pack in more nutrients than simple carbs because they are higher in fiber and digest more slowly. They help manage post-meal blood sugar spikes that are responsible for hyperactivity and poor concentration. Thus, it is also ideal for individuals with Type 2 Diabetes. Fiber and starch are the two types of complex carbohydrates. Fiber is especially important because it promotes bowel regularity and helps to control cholesterol. Starch is also found in some of the same foods as fiber. The difference is certain foods are considered more starchy than fibrous, such as potatoes.

Optimal Choices for complex carbohydrates

- *Fiber-rich grains*: Buckwheat, wild rice, barley, sorghum, quinoa (these are also rich in potassium, magnesium, and selenium).
- *Fiber-rich fruits*: Apples, berries, and bananas (avoid canned fruit because they usually contain added syrup).
- *Fiber-rich vegetables*: veggies play a pivotal role in overall health, eat broccoli, leafy greens, and carrots.
- *Nuts, Legumes & Seeds*: almonds, macadamia, flaxseeds, pumpkin seeds, lentils, kidney beans, chick peas, split peas, soy beans, pinto beans (these are good sources of folate, iron, and potassium).

Choosing the right carbs can take time and practice. It may take the help of your physician, holistic food practitioner, and/or registered dietician. Over time, with your own research, professional consultation and a careful eye for nutrition labels, you can start making healthier choices that will energize your body and protect your mental well-being.

Amino Acids

There are nine essential amino acids that perform a number of important and varied jobs in our bodies— mood, sleep, digestion, sexual function, and behavior. Let's take a look at the functions of each and the recommended food.

Optimal Choices for Amino Acids

- *Phenylalanine* is a precursor for the neurotransmitter's tyrosine, dopamine, epinephrine and norepinephrine. *Tyrosine* is an amino acid that is considered the building block of dopamine. This protein can get you feeling motivated!
    - Optimal choices with a good amount of phenylalanine, as well as tyrosine are soybeans, cheese, nuts, seeds, beef, lamb, chicken, pork, fish, eggs, dairy, beans and whole gains.

  Individuals suffering with Phenylketonuria should could their medical professional for personalized dietary intake. Keep in mind that artificial sweeteners contain phenylalanine and consuming large amounts of may lead to health complications. So, keep this mind, if mind when you're reaching for sweetener and consuming foods rich in phenylalanine.

- *Valine* is involved in energy production.
    - Optimal choices with good amount of this amino acid are beef, chicken, lamb, pork, fish, soybean, beans, nuts, seeds, and mushrooms.

- *Threonine* is involved in immune function and fat metabolism.
    - Optimal choices with good amount of this amino acid are lean beef, soy, pork, chicken, liver, cheese, shellfish, nuts, seeds, beans, and lentils.

- *Tryptophan* is a precursor to serotonin, which is involved in appetite, sleep and mood.
    - Optimal choices with good amount of this amino acid are salmon, chicken breast, eggs (boiled), spinach, seeds, milk, soy, and nuts.

- *Methionine* is involved in metabolism and detoxification.
    - Optimal choices with good amount of this amino acid are nuts, beef, lamb, cheese, turkey, pork, fish, shellfish, soy, eggs, dairy, and beans.

- *Leucine* is involved in regulating blood sugar levels.
    - Optimal choices with good amount of this amino acid are cheese, soybeans, beef, chicken, pork, nuts, seeds, fish, and beans.

- *Isoleucine* is involved in immune function and energy regulation.
    - Optimal choices with good amount of this amino acid are soybeans, cheese, beef, chicken, nuts, seeds, fish, and beans.

- *Lysine* is involved in energy production (motivation) and immune function.
    - Optimal choices with good amount of this amino acid are lean beef, cheese, turkey, chicken, pork, soy, fish, shrimp, shellfish, nuts, seeds, eggs, beans, and lentils.

- *Histidine* is involved in immune response, digestion, sexual function and sleep-wake cycles.
    - Optimal choices with good amount of this amino acid are beef, lamb, cheese, pork, chicken, turkey, soy, fish, nuts, seeds, eggs, beans, and whole grains.

As you may see, essential amino acids are pivotal to vital processes.

Vitamins and Minerals

Dietary nutrients are critical for brain structure and function, so they have a potentially profound impact on mental health. There is growing research that points out the detrimental effect of unhealthy diets and nutrient deficiencies. Likewise, research is pointing towards the protective value of a healthy diets for maintaining and promoting mental health. Most people think about the physical health benefits of vitamins and minerals, however deficiencies in these vital parts of your diet could worsen mood, anxiety, or thought processes.

B vitamins: B9 (Folate) and B12

We need B vitamins for a range of cellular and metabolic processes, and they have a critical role in the production of a range of brain chemicals. Although there are eight B vitamins, B9 (Folate) and B12 have been supported in research yet debated for their role in improving mental wellness. Folate (B9) deficiency has been linked to depressive mood. Studies report improvement in mood among people who respond poorly to antidepressants.

B12 deficiency can be overlooked due to its vagueness, meaning its symptoms can seem mundane—short attention span, low motivation, and lethargy. In extreme cases of B12 deficiency, symptoms ranged from hallucinations, irritability, thought fogginess, paranoia, memory loss, and depression. A deficiency can be detected through a blood panel ordered by your physician. B9 (Folate) and B12 can be acquired through whole food sources.

Vitamin D

Vitamin D is a fat-soluble compound that is pivotal to brain development as well as bone development. Studies have shown a link between pregnant mothers with low levels of vitamin D and increased schizophrenia risk for the unborn child (later in life), and a deficiency is linked to increased depressive symptoms (Anglin, 2003). Vitamin D can also be found in oily fish, fortified milk, and UVB-exposed mushrooms. You can make your own supply of vitamin D-enriched mushrooms by simply exposing them to sunlight. Get some sunshine for yourself! Vitamin D can be synthesized by sunlight. For 15 minutes each day, between 10am and 3pm, soak up some rays (recommended for summer, but for us who reside in sunny year-around places, it works wonders). Of course, proceed with caution if you have a family history of cancer or may be at risk of cancer due lifestyle habits.

Minerals

Minerals— zinc, magnesium and iron, have important roles in neurological function—learning and memory. Zinc is a rich trace mineral that is involved in many brain chemical reactions and supports good immune function. Deficiency in zinc has been linked depressive symptoms, specifically in major depressive disorder. Research has also shown that individuals with Alzheimer's had low levels of zinc. Magnesium is also involved in many brain chemistry reactions—calming the nervous system. Deficiency in magnesium has been linked to depressive systems, anxiety, poor attention, and hyperactivity. Iron is involved in several neurological activities—sex drive, motivation, and mood. Hence, an iron deficiency linked to depressive symptoms, anxiety, and developmental problems.

Optimal Choices Zinc:

Oysters, beef, chicken, tofu, pork, hemp seeds, nuts, lentils, yogurt, oatmeal, and mushrooms.

Optimal Choices Magnesium:

Avocados, bananas, dark chocolate, dark leafy greens, seeds, beans, fish, whole grains, nuts, and yogurt.

Optimal Choices Iron:

Beans, lentils, fortified cereals, beef, shellfish, dried fruit, dark leafy greens, dark chocolate, quinoa, mushrooms, and squash seeds.

Probiotics

Probiotics are neither vitamins nor minerals but plays an important role. Probiotics are live bacteria and yeasts that are referred to as "the good" microorganisms because they benefit the digestive system. Research shows a link between the bacteria in the gut and brain function, which affects mental health. When the structure of the gut microbiota, or the environment in stomach that supports bacteria, is less than optimal, it can cause an inflammatory response that may harm the nervous system. Specifically, harmful bacteria in the gastrointestinal (GI) tract can stimulate neural pathways and central nervous system (CNS), thus causing anxiety, poor concentration, and depression. Diets high in sugary, fatty and processed foods are associated with creating a harmful environment in the gut. A balanced microfloral environment, or gut environment with good bacteria is best supported by a diet high in the foods that nourish beneficial bacteria and reduce harmful microbial species, such as Helicobacter pylori.

Helicobacter pylori (H. pylori) is a type of bacteria that enters your body and live in your digestive tract. After H. pylori enters your body, it attacks the lining of your stomach, which usually protects you from the acid your body uses to digest food. Once the bacteria have done enough damage, acid can get through the lining, which leads to ulcers. These may bleed, cause infections, or keep food from moving through your digestive tract. Please do yourself a favor and keep that gut healthy! Dr. Peavy can attest to the mental anguish of several months and rounds of antibiotics to ease the discomfort of H. pylori.

Optimal Choices for Probiotics:
Fermented foods such as tempeh, sauerkraut, kimchi, kefir and yogurt, and pectin-rich foods such as fruit skin.

Water

So, you may be thinking, "Water, really?" But, yes! The lack of sufficient water intake causes dehydration and that has a significant impact on our mental well-being.

Dehydration and the Brain

There is a strong association between the amount of water in your body and brain function. Your brain can become inefficient when you are not drinking enough water. This can be attributed to salt and electrolytes, essential chemicals, not getting the minimum amount of hydration to remain effective. In turn, your cognitions, or ability to think becomes significantly impaired — poor memory, thought fogginess. Dehydration has been linked to increased pain sensitivity.

As discussed earlier in this chapter, the brain is made up of billions of microscopic cells and consists of approximately 60 percent water. The shape and structure of these cells are highly dependent on the amount water available. In order for minerals to travel to the brain, it need water to help it transport molecules to cells for proper function. When you become dehydrated, your brain compresses, or shrinks from the lack of water. This is a common source of headaches.

Dehydration and Mental Health

The brain cannot function at normal levels when there is not enough water intake. In fact, the brain's chemistry will be minimized, and mood will be profoundly affected. This will surely lead to clinical mental health concerns. The common symptoms of dehydration include anxiety, fatigue, and tension, which may lead to depression if symptoms are experienced for a prolonged period.

Everyday struggles will seem like a tug of war because dehydration impairs the ability to reason and concentrate. Thought fogginess will, surely, increase irritability and negativity. Digestive issues and pain sensitivity will further increase the level of stress that you are attempting to defeat. Furthermore, if you are presently taking prescribed medication to aid in stabilizing a mental health concerns, a lack of water in your body will have an impact on the medication's effectiveness. This is mainly because medication is activated in the body when it able to be properly broken down; hence, by water.

The public service announcements to "drink more water" is bigger than someone trying to control your body. It's about building a foundation to help manage physical and mental health. The recommended water intake is 3.7 liters (15 cups) for the average adult male and 2.7 liters (11 cups) for the average adult female. Make sure it's purified, alkaline, or spring water.

Table 3. Summary of Nutrient Deficiency

Nutrient	Deficiency Effects	Avoid	Consume
Essential Fatty Acids	-Poor Attention -Neurological problems -Low Mood -Worsened psychosis	Sugar Fast Food (Fried) Processed Foods Alcohol	Salmon, chicken breasts, acai, pistachios, grapeseed oil, black seed oil
Complex "Carbs" Carbohydrates	-Poor Concentration -Hyperactivity	Sugary foods and drinks	Apples, bananas, green leafy veggies
Amino Acids	-Low Mood -Sleep Disturbance -Feelings of Uneasiness -Sex Drive	Sugar Fast Food (Fried) Processed Foods Alcohol	Avocado, Eggs, Cheese, Fish Turkey, lentils, mushrooms, soy
Vitamins & Minerals (Including Probiotics)	-Irritability -Anxiety -Low Mood -Confusion -Psychosis	Sugar Fast Food (Fried) Processed Foods Alcohol	Oysters, beef, chicken, tofu, avocados, bananas, quinoa, mushrooms
Water	-Foggy Thinking -Anxiety -Tiredness -Tension	Sweetened/Flavored Water	Alkaline Water Spring Water Filtered Water

Chapter 3

Depression

"There are wounds that never show on the body that are deeper and more hurtful than anything that bleeds." ~ Laurell K. Hamilton

Understanding Depressive Symptoms

Feelings of sadness and grief are normal emotional responses. At some point in our lives, we all experience those feelings, but they typically dissipate after a few days. For example, an individual might feel sad (up to nearly two weeks) after the loss of a loved one which may be accompanied by crying and slight sleep disturbance, but they are able to manage their day-to-day. When those days turn into two weeks or more, it may be a major depressive episode, or clinically known as major depressive disorder (major depression). Major depression is a diagnosable condition that is characterized by feelings of worthlessness or guilt, poor concentration, loss of energy, fatigue, thoughts of suicide or preoccupation with death, loss or increase of appetite and weight, a disturbed sleep pattern, slowing down or low motivation (both physically and mentally), agitation (restlessness or anxiety). For example, an individual experiences increased sadness for two months following a divorce or breakup; they have gradually isolated themselves, no longer find interests in favorite hobbies, and has trouble managing their day-to-day.

Depressive Episodes in the United States

In the United States, there was an estimated 16.2 million adults who experienced at least one major depressive episode in year 2016. Of those episodes, occurrences among women were higher (8.5%) as compared to men (4.8%). There were an estimated 2.2 million adolescents aged 12-17 who had at least one major depressive episode with severe impairment; representing nearly 70%. Nearly 3.1 million adolescents aged 12-17 had at least one major depressive episode without severe impairment; representing nearly 13%. Of the combined episodes of depression among adolescents, occurrences among girls were higher (19.4%) as compared to boys (6.4%).

Links to Depressive Symptoms

So, you may ask yourself, "What causes depression"? Biologically, depression occurs when there is an abnormal excess or inhibition of signals in the brain that control mood, thinking, pain, and other sensory stimulation. Both neurotransmitters, dopamine and serotonin, are believed to play a role in depression. Dopamine is responsible for motivation and reward— pleasure, satisfaction, and hopefulness. Do remember you remember how you felt when you finally accomplished that goal, earned or won a prize? Or maybe, listening to music by a phenomenal band such as Tank and The Bangas? It is the transmission of dopamine in the brain that allows us to find pleasure. If you think of the urban term, "dope", which describes the highest feeling of pleasure; this may help you remember to role of dopamine. Learning something new is dope! In depression, a dopamine dysfunction (caused by short or long-term stress, pain, or trauma) is linked to low motivation, helplessness, and loss of interest in our favorite things. Serotonin is involved in how we process emotions and sleep. Diets high in sugary, fatty and processed foods are associated with creating harmful bacteria in the gut. This can cause inflammation and trigger neurotransmitters, thus causing depressive symptoms.

Treatment:

Depression can be assessed and diagnosed by medical and mental health professionals. The following are current treatments for mood, specifically depression:

- *Cognitive-Behavioral Therapy (CBT)* is therapy whereby the therapist helps you to identify negative thought patterns as well as your behavioral responses to stressful and challenging situations. It is proven to be a highly effective form of treatment. In some cases, if more intensive treatment is needed, CBT will still be used in conjunction with other treatments.

- *Antidepressants* are prescribed medications that are used to help correct abnormal neurotransmitter activity.

- *Transcranial magnetic stimulation (TMS)* uses a magnet similar in strength to that used in a magnetic resonance imaging (MRI) machine. TMS is used to stimulate nerve cells in the area of the brain thought to control mood. These magnetic pulses may have a positive effect on the brain's neurotransmitter levels, making long-term remission possible. This treatment is used for severe depressive disorders.

Optimal Nutritional Suggestions:

As with any treatment, nutrition plays a vital role in our mental well-being. We learned earlier, there are certain deficiencies in neurotransmitters (dopamine and serotonin), and nutrients (Zinc, Magnesium, Iron) that have been linked to disturbances in mood. Let's take a look at food and herbs that contain the protective properties of nutrients that can help combat depressive and other mood disturbances.

Herbs

- Oregano
- Pepperwort
- Thyme
- Linden flower
- Lavender
- Turmeric
- Damiana
- Wild Bergamot
- Sage
- Dill
- Rosemary
- Maca (Lepidium meyenii)
- Maidenhair tree (Ginkgo biloba)
- Chamomile
- Grapeseed oil
- Black seed oil

Foods

- Cold water high-fat fish (wild Alaskan salmon, sardines, anchovies, mackerel, shad, herring, and trout)
- Poultry (Turkey and chicken breasts
- Shellfish (shrimp, lobster, oysters)
- Tofu
- Probiotic-rich foods (Plain yogurt, Sauerkraut, Kimchi and Fermented soy products)

- Dark green leafy vegetables (swiss chard, kale, spinach, purslane, mustard greens, and collards)
- Mushrooms
- Dark chocolate
- Watermelon
- Lemons
- Lentils
- Acai, elderberry
- pistachios
- Pumpkin Seeds
- Brazil Nuts
- Almonds

Water

The recommended water intake is 3.7 liters (15 cups) for the average adult male and 2.7 liters (11 cups) for the average adult female. As discussed in Chapter 2, the consumption caffeine, sugary drinks, and alcohol causes dehydration. This means that more water will be required to remove these substances from your body. Research has found that various drinks can take the body up to 3 times the amount of water to process that drink. For example, consumption of a 12 oz. beer will take your body 36 ounces of water to flush out that one can of beer. Also, it is important to note that water intake will vary due to certain medical problems such as renal failure and congestive heart failure. If you have any medical conditions or prescribed medication, please consult your physician and/or a dietician for the recommended water intake.

It recommended that you consume filtered-water, i.e. spring water, alkaline water, or distilled water. It is not recommended to drink unknown water sources or tap water as some municipal water systems contain traces of lead which lead-filled water is known to cause neurological damage that is linked to depression. Don't like the taste of water? Well, add a little lemon or lime. Maybe, consider unsweetened carbonated water with a squeeze of lime. It's a better choice than drinking pop.

Mind, Body & Earth Suggestions:

➤ Exercise can have antidepressant effects. It doesn't matter what type of physical activity as long as you get moving for at least 30 minutes for three to five days per week. Here's a few ideas for any fitness level:
  o Mindfulness Walk:
    While walking outdoors, make it your duty to aware of your body. Start by noticing how your body feels and moves with each step. Simply, heighten your awareness of your environment by noting what you see, hear, smell, and feel. Additionally, the sunlight provides the Vitamin D needed.
  o Yoga:
    If you haven't practiced before, it can seem intimidating. A great way to start, is watching YouTube videos and start practicing at home until you're ready to join a yoga class.

➤ Visualization. It uses the power of the mind to create positive emotions. You simply, imagine a relaxing scene in detail. Don't under estimate the power of your mind. What you create, it shall be! It's great for anxiety, too!

➤ Here are a few crystals that help with mood: Botswana Agate, Smokey Quartz, Sunstone, Lepidolite, and Amethyst.

SMOKED SALMON FRITTATAS

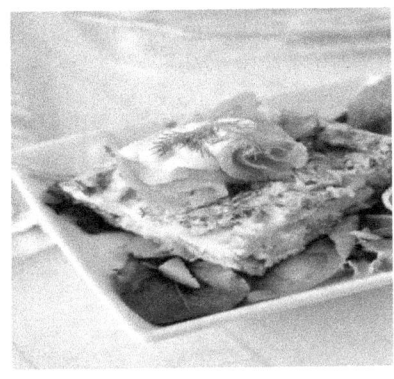

This tasty dish is a great source of serotonin boosting power. Frittatas are great dish to start breakfast or brunch.

Ingredients (Serves 6)

- 1 tablespoon olive oil
- 1/2 cup chopped red onion
- 4 ounces smoked salmon, roughly chopped
- 1 tablespoon capers
- 1 ½ cups egg substitute
- 1/4 cup 2% milk
- 1/4 teaspoon sea salt
- 1/4 teaspoon freshly cracked black pepper
- 1 (3-ounce) of cottage cheese
- 1 tablespoon chopped chives

Instructions

1. Preheat the oven to 350°F.
2. Heat olive oil in an 8-inch oven-proof sauté pan over medium heat. Add onion and cook until translucent but not brown, about 4 minutes. Add the salmon and capers and cook 1 minute, stirring occasionally.
3. Whisk eggs, milk, salt, and pepper until well beaten. Pour over salmon and stir gently with a rubber spatula,

30 seconds. Scatter cream cheese over the top and cook, without stirring, until the edges appear firm, about 3 minutes.
4. Transfer skillet to oven and bake until nicely browned and puffed, about 20 minutes.
5. To serve, invert onto a serving plate, cut into squares and top with a thin slice of smoked salmon and chopped chives, dill, or your favorite garnish.

LAVENDER LEMONADE

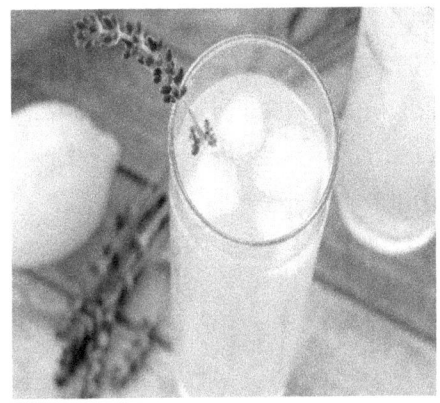

This refreshing drink is a good source of dopamine balancing, GABA. This twist on an old-fashioned favorite is excellent for mood imbalances such as depression (including anxiety, restlessness and insomnia).

Ingredients (Serves 2-4)

- 1 cup maple syrup
- 5 cups of water
- ¼ cup dried lavender
- 6 lemons

Instructions

1. Boil dried lavender and maple syrup half the water. Let steep for 20 mins.
2. Strain mixture and pour into a larger carafe or container.
3. Juice 5 lemons and add lemon juice to the carafe with remaining water. Add sliced lemons. Slice the remaining 1 lemon and put to the side for garnish. Chill and serve.

WATERMELON WITH DILL

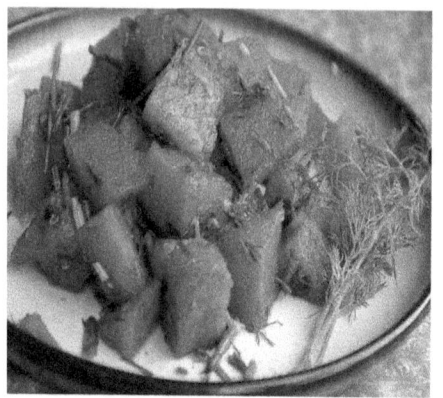

This refreshing snack is a good source of dopamine and serotonin. This twist on favorite is excellent for mood imbalances such as depression (including anxiety).

Ingredients (Servings vary)

- 1 cup of seeded watermelon
- Fresh Dill
- Pinch of sea salt (optional)

Instructions

1. Place chunks of seeded watermelon in bowl and sprinkle dill over top. (Optional: You may add a pinch of sea salt. This creates a salty sweet contrast that allows the sweetness of the melon to stand out.)
2. Now, eat and enjoy!

Chapter 4

Stress and Anxiety

"Worrying doesn't take away tomorrow's troubles; it takes away today's peace".
~Author Unknown

Understanding Stress

Everyone feels stressed from time to time. Stress is a physical and emotional reaction that people experience as they encounter changes in life. Some people may cope with stress more effectively or recover from stressful events more quickly than others. There are different types of stress—all of which carry physical and mental health risks. A stressor may be a one time or short-term occurrence, or it can be an occurrence that keeps happening over a long period of time.

Examples of stress include:

- Routine stress related to the pressures of work, school, family and other daily responsibilities
- Stress brought about by a sudden negative change, such as losing a job, divorce, or illness
- Traumatic stress experienced in an event like a major accident, war, assault, or a natural disaster where people may be in danger of being seriously hurt or killed. People who experience traumatic stress often experience temporary symptoms of mental illness, but most recover naturally soon after.

Stress and Health Implications

Stress is a normal feeling. However, long-term stress may contribute to or worsen a range of health problems including digestive disorders, headaches, sleep disorders, and other symptoms. Stress may worsen asthma and has been linked to depression, anxiety, and other mental illnesses.

Health problems can occur if the stress response goes on for too long or becomes chronic, such as when the source of stress is constant, or if the response continues after the danger has subsided. With chronic stress, those same life-saving responses in your body can suppress immune, digestive, sleep, and reproductive systems, which may cause them to stop working normally. Different people may feel stress in different ways. For example, some people experience mainly digestive symptoms, while others may have headaches, sleeplessness, sadness, anger or irritability. People under chronic stress are prone to more frequent and severe viral infections, such as the flu or common cold.

Stress can motivate people to prepare or perform, like when they need to take a test or interview for a new job. Stress can even be life-saving in some situations. In response to danger, your body prepares to face a threat or flee to safety. In these situations, your pulse quickens, you breathe faster, your muscles tense, your brain uses more oxygen and increases activity — all functions aimed at survival.

Routine stress may be the hardest type of stress to notice at first. Because the source of stress tends to be more constant than in cases of acute or traumatic stress, the body gets no clear signal to return to normal functioning. Over time, continued strain on your body from routine stress may contribute to serious health problems, such as heart disease, high blood pressure, diabetes, and other illnesses, as well as mental disorders like depression or anxiety.

TABLE 4. Common Symptoms in Domains of Anxiety

Physical	Psychological	Behavioral
• **Cardiovascular** rapid heart rate, heart pounding, pain in chest • **Gastrointestinal** diarrhea, vomiting, nausea, choking • **Musculoskeletal** Muscle aches in neck, shoulders, or back; restlessness, trembles • **Neurological** light-headedness, headache, numbness, sweating • **Respiratory** shortness of breath, hyperventilation	• Racing thoughts • Poor concentration • Poor memory • Fatigue • Feeling on Edge • Sleep Disturbance • Intense Dreams • Excessive and/or unrealistic fear and worry about past and/or future.	• Preoccupations and/or strong impulses to perform a task • Avoidant of situations • Anguish in social situations • Extreme Fear with specificity (e.g. spiders, heights, etc.)

Understanding Anxiety

Everyone experiences anxiety at multiple points in their lives. The utility of anxiety can help a person navigate dangerous situations and be the core of motivation in problem-solving. The experience of anxiety may come in varying degrees of severity ranges from a terrifying panic attacks to mild nervousness. Likewise, anxiety can vary in how long it lasts, from minutes to years. There are distinctions between normal anxiety and anxiety disorder; anxiety disorders are more intense, longs lasting, and interferes with a person's interpersonal and work relationships.

The symptoms of anxiety encompass three domains: physical (effecting heart, stomach, muscles, brain, and lungs), psychological (effecting thoughts, memory, sleep, and worry) and behavioral (obsessions, avoidance, and strong fear responses). Common symptoms of anxiety can be found in anxiety disorders. Table 4 provides a comprehensive list of symptoms that are found in each of the domains.

Anxiety in the United States

In the United States, there is an estimated 40 million, or 18.1 % (NIH, 2016) adults age 18 or order who experienced an anxiety disorder in a given year. Yet, making it the most common mental illness in the United States; treated and untreated. In fact, anxiety disorders are greatly treatable, however only less than 40% of those living in distress receive treatment. Research has shown that 54 % of woman and 46 % of men experience an anxiety disorder. Individuals with an anxiety disorder are more likely to frequent their doctors and more likely to be treated inpatient for psychiatric disorders than individuals who do not have an anxiety disorder.

Anxiety may be experienced in various ways. The specific types of anxiety disorders include separation anxiety disorder, selective mutism, specific phobia, social phobia, panic disorder, agoraphobia, and generalized anxiety disorder. This includes obsessive-compulsive disorders such as obsessive-compulsive disorder, body dysmorphic disorder, hoarding disorder, trichotillomania, and excoriation disorder and trauma-stress related disorders, such as reactive attachment disorder, disinhibited social engagement disorder, post-traumatic stress disorder (PTSD), acute stress disorder, and adjustment disorder. In this book we will not cover each of those disorders separately, however, we will focus on the common symptoms of anxiety as seen in Table 4.

Links to Anxiety

So, you may be attempting to figure out, "Why am I so darn anxious?" Anxiety disorders develop from a complex set of risk factors, including genetics, brain chemistry, personality, and life events. Anxiety is chiefly triggered by perceived threats in the environment, however some people are more susceptible to respond with anxiety when threatened due to higher risk factors.

Risk Factors

Let's take a look at this example. Clarissa's husband filed for divorce after 17 years of marriage. Gradually, Clarissa begins to feel as if things are following apart. She has increasingly grown fearful of her parents dying, her children being taken away, and even intruding thoughts of losing her job. Clarissa's inability to perform her work and home duties are impaired due to headaches, inability to focus, and constant stomach pains. This is an example how anxiety has manifested in Clarissa's life. The cause is not only the major life stressor—divorce. There are other risk factors that have contributed to how she is handling the life change, such as being a woman, the trauma of her parent's "bitter" divorce when she was 11 years old, and her family history of anxiety disorders.

Here's a snapshot of risk factors that make it likely to respond with anxiety:

- Being female (more reported cases from women)
- Sensitive emotional nature, tending to see the world as threatening
- Alcohol Abuse
- Traumatic Experiences
- History of anxiety in youth, including shyness

Family factors can increase this risk:

- Family history of anxiety disorders
- Parents with history of alcohol abuse
- Divorce and separation
- Poverty, presently or history of
- Childhood of any forms of abuse (physical, emotional, sexual or neglect)

Medical factors can increase this risk:

- Prescription drugs side effects
- Intoxication with alcohol, amphetamines, caffeine, marijuana, cocaine, inhalants, and hallucinogens.
- Withdrawal from alcohol, sedatives, cocaine and anxiety medications (That is correct! People can

experience withdrawal from prescription anxiety medications.).
- Medical conditions such as Vitamin B12 deficiency, cardiac problems (arrhythmias), respiratory problems (chronic obstructive pulmonary disease), and hyperthyroidism.

Food Biology of Anxiety

When we examine food's role in anxiety, we are taking a look at how these foods affect the brain. As mentioned in Chapter 2, production of GABA is decreased when consuming foods high in sugar, which causes an increase in excitability. Stress can contribute to memory loss. Specifically, cortisol damage brain cells in the hippocampus causing poor memory and cognitive impairment. Additionally, dehydration can cause anxiousness. Alcohol can have a negative impact on hydration and sleep, both of which can trigger anxiety symptom. Alcohol changes levels of serotonin and the neurotransmitters in the brain, which worsens anxiety and when the alcohol tapers off, it may increase anxiety. High doses of caffeine can cause the unpleasant effects anxiety and nervousness. Be mindful before you place an order for a "grande" cup of coffee!

Treatment:

Stress and anxiety can be assessed and diagnosed by medical and mental health professionals. The following are current treatments for anxiety (and stress as by-product), specifically depression:

> ➤ ***Cognitive-Behavioral Therapy (CBT)*** is therapy whereby the therapist helps you to identify negative

thought patterns as well as your behavioral responses to stressful and challenging situations. It is proven to be a highly effective form of treatment.

> *Antidepressants* are prescribed medications that are used to help correct abnormal neurotransmitter activity.

> *Benzodiazepines* are anti-anxiety medications that are effective but highly addictive, sedative, damaging to memory, and has rebound anxiety (meaning that it's likely that you develop worsened anxiety as result of stopping medication). Co-author, Dr. Peavy reports assessing and admitting dozens of people into inpatient hospitalization detox and substance abuse programs for addiction to benzodiazepines.

Optimal Nutritional Suggestions:

As with any treatment, nutrition plays a vital role in our mental well-being. We learned earlier, there are certain deficiencies in neurotransmitters (serotonin and GABA), and nutrients (magnesium, complex carbohydrates, B12, probiotic, and water) that have been linked to stress and anxiety. Let's take a look at food and herbs that contain the protective properties of nutrients that can help combat stress and anxiety.

Herbs
- Blue Vervain
- Prodigiosa
- Bugleweed
- Linden
- Valerian
- Lavender

- Lemon Balm
- Tumeric
- Cinnamon
- Damiana
- Green Tea
- Cilantro

- Chamomile
- Passion Flower
- Kava kava
- Ashwagandha
- Rhodiola

Foods

- Cold water high-fat fish (wild Alaskan salmon, sardines, anchovies, mackerel, shad, herring, and trout)
- Turkey
- Eggs
- Tofu
- Cheese
- Probiotic-rich foods (Plain yogurt, Sauerkraut, and Kimchi)
- Dark Green vegetables (Spinach and Swiss chard)
- Dark chocolate
- Pineapple
- Bananas
- Oats
- Pumpkin Seeds
- Brazil Nuts
- Almond

Water

The recommended water intake is 3.7 liters (15 cups) for the average adult male and 2.7 liters (11 cups) for the average adult female. As discussed in Chapter 2, the consumption caffeine, sugary drinks, and alcohol causes dehydration which, literally puts a squeeze on the brain. This leads to inability to concentrate and feelings of nervousness. The body will have to work hard to flush out those substances, which can only be accomplished with increased water intake. As mentioned in Chapter 3, various drinks can take the body up to 3 times the amount of water (based on the ounces of beverage you have consumed) to process that particularly drink. Again, it is important to note that water intake will vary due to certain medical problems such as renal failure and congestive heart failure. If you have any medical conditions or prescribed medication, please consult your physician and/or a dietician for the recommended water intake.

It is recommended that you consume filtered-water, i.e. spring water, alkaline water, distilled water, etc. It is not recommended to drink unknown water sources or tap water from some municipal water systems because it may contain traces of lead, which lead-filled water is known to cause neurological damage that is linked to depression. If you do not like the state of water, start by adding the juice from a citrus fruit. Also, consider unsweetened carbonated water with a squeeze of lime. It's a better choice than drinking pop.

Mind, Body & Earth Suggestions:
- Exercise produce endorphins (chemicals in the brain that act as natural painkillers). About five minutes of aerobic exercise can begin to stimulate anti-anxiety effects. It doesn't matter what type of physical activity as long as you get moving for at least 30 minutes for three to five days per week. Here's a few ideas for any fitness level:
    - Fitness Class:
      There are too many to name, but here's a few that we like: Zumba, Hip-Hop Aerobics, Cross-fit, and Kickboxing.
    - Dance:

Yes, we said dance! Turn on "dance" or "party" music and get that body moving for 30-45 minutes.

- Deep Breathing. It is an excellent and discreet way to managing emotions such as stress and anxiety.
    - Sit comfortably and place one hand on your abdomen. Breathe in through your nose, deeply enough that the hand on your abdomen rises. Hold the air in your lungs, and then exhale slowly through your mouth, with your lips puckered as if you are blowing through a straw. The KEY is to go slow: Time the inhalation (4s), pause (4s), and exhalation (6s). Practice for 3 to 5 minutes
- Grab crayons and map pencils! Coloring (and drawing) works wonders for managing stress and anxiety, and depression, too! Grab a mandala coloring page, coloring book, or plain paper and start releasing those negative feelings.
- Try wearing natural stones with healing properties for anxiety. Here are a few that we suggest: Clear Quartz, Amethyst, Rose Quartz, Citrine, Black Tourmaline or Aventurine.

BAKED TURKEY WITH SAUTEED COLLARD GREENS

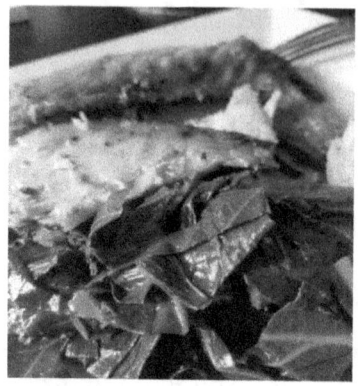

This is southern comfort at its finest. Turkey has the amino acid, tryptophan, and collards have beta-carotene, vitamin E, and Omega 3 to help boost antioxidant levels.... making this a powerful anti-anxiety meal with the added benefit to but you asleep.

Baked Turkey Wings

Ingredients (Serves 2-4)

- 4 turkey wings
- 1 tablespoon olive oil or coconut oil
- 1 teaspoon minced garlic
- 1 teaspoon of turmeric
- ½ cup of chopped onion
- 1 teaspoon of cracked black pepper
- 1 ½ cups water, divided
- 1 teaspoon of sea salt (optional)

Instructions

1. Preheat oven to 350 degrees F (175 degrees C).
2. Place turkey wings and onion in a casserole dish. Sprinkle sea salt, turmeric, black pepper, and garlic on both sides of each wing. Pour 1/2 cup water into the casserole dish. Cover casserole dish.
3. Bake in the preheated oven until browned, 1 hour. Pour remaining 1 cup water and continue until tender, 1 hour.

Sautéed Collard Greens

Ingredients (Serves 2-4)

- 2 tablespoons extra-virgin olive oil
- 6 garlic cloves, thinly sliced
- ¼ teaspoon crushed red-pepper flakes
- ½ cup of raw chopped red bell peppers (optional)
- 2 heads collard greens (about 1 pound each), tough stems and ribs removed, leaves coarsely chopped
- Sea salt
- ½ cup water

Instructions

1. Heat oil in a large sauté pan over medium heat.
2. Cook garlic, stirring often, until golden, about 3 minutes. Stir in red-pepper flakes, and cook until fragrant, about 30 seconds. Stir in collard greens and 1 teaspoon salt. (Optional: add in chopped red bell pepper)
3. Reduce heat to medium-low. Add water, and steam, covered, until greens are just tender, and water evaporates, about 10 minutes. If greens are ready but there is still water in the pan, raise heat to medium-high, and cook, uncovered, until completely evaporated.

BANANA OAT BERRY SMOOTHIE

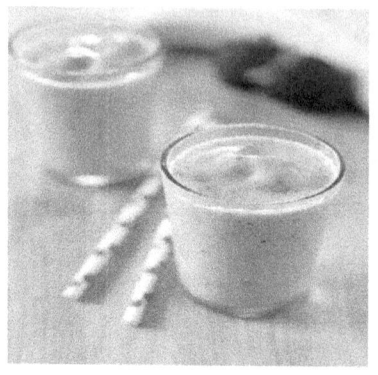

This delicious treat in a glass is packed with probiotics, magnesium, and zinc to give you the serotonin and GABA boost needed to decrease anxiety.

Ingredients (Serves 1-2)

- 1/2 cup unsweetened yogurt
- 1 large banana
- 1 cup of frozen strawberries
- 1 Orange (remove peel)
- 1 cup oats (raw or cooked)
- ½ cup of purified water

Instructions

1. Pour yogurt and strawberries into blender. Blend until smooth.
2. Add oats, peeled orange, and ½ cup of water. Blend until smooth.
3. Now, add banana. Blend until smooth.
4. Enjoy your delicious smoothie!

Chapter 5

Attention Deficit and Hyperactivity

"I wish I could sleep but my ADD kicks in and...one sheep, two sheep, cow, turtle, duck, old McDonald had a farm...hey Macarena"
~ malikovadarya.info

Understanding Attention Deficit-Hyperactivity Disorder

Kimberly is trying her hardest to listen and wait her turn to speak during conversation but, she quickly interrupts the other speaker to make her point. This could be interpreted by the speaker as rude and it could have lasting negative consequences. John is tasked with paying attention in an important meeting, when he suddenly realizes that he has missed valuable information because he began to daydream during the presentation. John's inability to recap information from the presentation, could be interpreted as disinterest and could offend to presenter. Can you relate to either or both situations? Both situations can be distressing for individuals. Well, this is the experience of a person dealing with Attention Deficit – Hyperactivity Disorder (ADHD).

ADHD can damage professional and personal relationships as well as self-esteem. Inattentive symptoms can lead to poor organization, difficulty completing tasks, and forgetting responsibilities. Hyperactive symptoms can cause impulsive decision-making, a persistent need for stimulation, and thrill-seeking. According to The American Psychiatric Association (DSM-5, 2013), ADHD is defined as a persistent pattern of inattention, hyperactivity, and/or impulsivity that impedes functioning or development. Let's take a look at the three distinctions that characterize ADHD.

- Inattentiveness appears when a person has difficulty sustaining focus, experiences disorganization, meanders off task, and lacks persistence. It must be noted that these problems are not due to rebelliousness or lack of comprehension.
- Hyperactivity appears when a person excessively fidgets, taps, or talks and/or has difficulty being still during appropriate times (restlessness).
- Impulsivity appears when a person makes hasty decisions without well-thought out plans and demonstrates difficulty to delay gratification. These characteristics are associated with a person demonstrating socially intrusive behaviors such as interrupting others.

Keeping in mind the aforementioned distinctions, attention deficit-hyperactivity disorder (ADHD) is diagnosed according to the presence of inattention, hyperactivity, and impulsivity. ADHD is a developmental disorder that begins in childhood (before age 12), however it is possible to receive this diagnosis as late as adolescence or adulthood. Specially, symptoms are believed to first appear between the ages of 3-6 but are commonly diagnosed around age 7. In order to receive a diagnosis of ADHD, a person must have at least five symptoms of inattentive, and/or hyperactivity-impulsivity that are present in two or more settings (such as home, work, or school) and there must be evidence that the symptoms significantly impact the person's functioning in these settings. In it important to keep in mind, that not everyone who experiences inattentiveness and/or hyperactivity has been diagnosed. Therefore, we will explore the symptoms (inattentiveness, impulsivity, and hyperactivity) and foods that help.

ADHD in the United States

According the American Psychiatric Association (DSM-5, 2013), 5% of U.S. children have ADHD, which other studies in the United States have estimated higher rates in community samples. Over 4 % of American adults over the age of 18 attempt to cope with ADHD on a daily basis. Research has shown that males are almost three times more likely to be diagnosed with ADHD than females. During their lifetimes, 12.9 percent of men will be diagnosed with disorder that affects attention and 4.9 percent of women will be diagnosed. Nearly 50 % of adults with ADHD also struggle with anxiety disorders.

Links to Inattentiveness and Hyperactivity

It is not known what causes a person to have ADHD, but some researchers have looked at a neurotransmitters, dopamine and serotonin as possible contributors to inattentiveness, impulsivity, and hyperactivity. Lower levels of dopamine are associated problems paying attention. Dopamine allows us to regulate emotional responses and take action to achieve specific rewards, but it does not account for dysregulation of emotion--impulse control and aggression. Thus, lower levels of serotonin are associated with impulsive and aggressive behavior.

Food Biology of ADHD (inattentive, impulsive, hyperactive behavior)

When we examine food's role in ADHD, we are taking a look at how these foods affect the brain. As mentioned in Chapter 2, complex carbohydrates help regulate blood sugar (insulin) spikes after a meal which is responsible for hyperactivity and poor concentration. Serotonin is not found in foods, but tryptophan, that key amino acid, is. If you combine high-tryptophan foods with complex carbohydrates, you will get a serotonin boost. Fiber and starch are the two types of complex carbohydrates. However, if you consume simple carbohydrates such as raw sugar, brown sugar, corn syrup and high-fructose corn syrup, glucose, fructose, and sucrose, or fruit juice concentrate; it will decrease ability to pay attention and cause hyperactive behavior. Harmful bacteria in gut can cause inflammation and fuel neurotransmitters, thus causing poor concentration. Diets high in sugary, fatty and processed foods are associated with creating a harmful environment in the gut. Likewise, production of GABA is decreased when consuming foods high in sugar, which causes an increase hyperactive and impulsive behavior. Alcohol can have a negative impact on hydration and sleep, both of which can trigger anxiety symptom. Alcohol changes levels of serotonin and the neurotransmitters in the brain, which worsens impulsive behavior. We shouldn't have to repeat this one, but, lack of proper water intake can worsen symptoms.

Treatment:

Problems with poor attention, impulsive behavior, or hyperactive behavior (ADHD) can be assessed and diagnosed by medical and mental health professionals. The following are current treatments for ADHD:

> *Psychotherapy* for ADHD focuses learning personalized coping skills. This achieved through education about ways to reduce symptoms, skill building, and identifying strengths and weaknesses.

> *Stimulants* are prescribed medications that are used to help correct abnormal neurotransmitter activity.

Optimal Nutritional Suggestions:

As with any treatment, nutrition plays a vital role in our mental well-being. We learned earlier, there are certain deficiencies in neurotransmitters (serotonin and dopamine), and nutrients (essential fatty acids, complex carbohydrates, B12, and probiotic) that have been linked to inattentive, impulsive, and hyperactive behavior associated with ADHD. Let's take a look at food and herbs that contain the protective properties of nutrients that can help combat these symptoms.

Herbs

- Rosemary
- Nutmeg
- Damiana
- Peppermint
- Ginseng (Red Ginseng)
- Rhodiola rosea
- Avena sativa
- Gotu kola (Centella asiatica)
- Brahmi (Bacopa monnieri)

Foods

- Cold water high-fat fish (wild Alaskan salmon, sardines, anchovies, mackerel, shad, herring, and trout)
- Shellfish (shrimp, lobster, oysters, crab)
- Eggs
- Cheese
- Probiotic-rich foods (Plain yogurt,

- Sauerkraut, and Kimchi)
- Cabbage
- Celery
- Broccoli
- Cauliflower
- Carrots
- Pineapple
- Fiber-rich fruits (apples, strawberries, blueberries, raspberries and bananas)
- Legumes (lentils, kidney beans, chick peas, split peas, soy beans, pinto beans)
- Fiber-rich grains (buckwheat, wild rice, barley, sorghum, quinoa)
- Nuts (walnuts and brazil nuts)
- Omega-3 EFA oil (Flaxseed or hempseed)
- Seeds (chia, hemp, pumpkin, and sesame)
- Mango
- Coconut

Water

Yep, and again! The recommended water intake is 3.7 liters (15 cups) for the average adult male and 2.7 liters (11 cups) for the average adult female. As we learned in this chapter, consumption caffeine, sugary drinks, and alcohol not increasing causes one to be distracted but, as discussed in other chapters it causes dehydration which, literally puts a squeeze on the brain leading to poor concentration and feelings of nervousness. Now, imagine the impact of those combined. Yikes!

Mind, Body & Earth Suggestions:

➢ We know this already! Exercise produce endorphins. Anything that gets your heart pounding— like aerobic exercise is key. Here's a few ideas for any fitness level:

   o Heart pounding activities:

- Running
- Walking briskly
- Biking
- Swimming laps
- Boxing

  o Mind-Heart challenging activities:
  - Yoga
  - Rock climbing

➢ Deep Breathing. Get oxygen flowing for more focus!

  o Sit comfortably and place one hand on your abdomen. Breathe in through your nose, deeply enough that the hand on your abdomen rises. Hold the air in your lungs, and then exhale slowly through your mouth, with your lips creased as if you are blowing through a straw. The KEY is to go slow: Time the inhalation (4s), pause (4s), and exhalation (6s). Practice for 3 to 5 minutes.

➢ Here are a few natural crystals with healing properties to calm the mind and help with concentration: Amazonite, Amethyst, Hematite, and Lepidolite

FRUITY YOGURT CUP

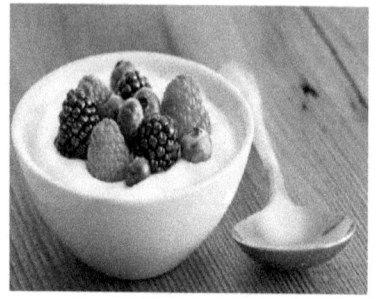

This simple treat is what you need to get your day started with focus. It is great for breakfast or snack.

Ingredients (Serves 1)

- 1/2 cup unsweetened yogurt
- 1 large banana
- 1 handful of strawberries and blueberries

Instructions

1. Start by cleaning berries of pesticides. Fill a large bowl with 4 parts water to 1 part plain white vinegar. Soak the berries in the mixture for 20 minutes. Then rise.
2. Pour yogurt and banana into blender. Blend until smooth.
3. Place blended yogurt into bowl and top with strawberries and blueberries.
4. Enjoy your delicious smoothie!

ROSEMARY LEMON CHICKEN

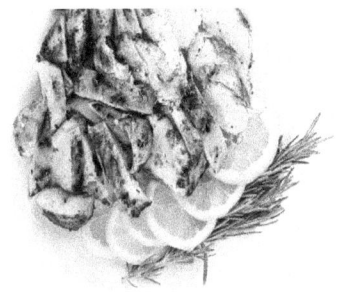

Rosemary lemon chicken is a favorite that the whole family can enjoy. It's packed with protein, vitamins, and minerals needed to keep you focused!

Ingredients (Serves 4)

- pound skinless, boneless chicken breast
- 2 tablespoons coconut oil
- ¼ cup lemon juice
- 2 cloves garlic, pressed
- ¼ cup fresh rosemary, minced
- ½ teaspoon sea salt
- 4 cups of any vegetable from list

Instructions

1. In a medium bowl, combine olive oil, lemon juice, garlic, rosemary and salt
2. Rinse chicken breasts, pat dry and place in an 7 x 11 inch baking dish
3. Pour marinade over chicken, cover and refrigerate for at least 30 minutes or up to 6 hours
4. Heat grill and cook chicken for 5-7 minutes per side until browned and cooked in the center
5. Add grilled vegetables from list.
6. Serve and Enjoy!

Chapter 6

Cognitive Decline

"Please remember the real me when I cannot remember you"
~Mountain Wisdom

Understanding Cognitive Decline

Everyone forgets things at times, right? How often have you misplaced your car keys or the remote control? What about the "tip of my tongue" moment, but you just couldn't remember the name? As we age, it is quite common to have some degree of memory problems and a modest decline in our thinking faculties. Though, there is a difference between normal changes in memory and the cognitive decline associated with Alzheimer's and related disorders.

Cognitive decline is described as memory loss in which a person experiences an abnormal level of forgetfulness and inability to recall past events in their life. A person who is experiencing cognitive decline may have difficulty learning, using language, or remembering things. In other words, the brain does not work as well as it did in the past. It's not common for normal age-related memory loss to prevent someone from living a full, productive life. Depression, anxiety, and stress has been linked to memory problems, such as forgetfulness or confusion. There can be difficulty to focus on work or other tasks, make decisions, or think clearly. It is often associated with short-term memory loss. For instance, you might occasionally forget a person's name, but recall it later in the day. You might misplace something important but can retrace your steps to find it.

Cognitive decline can be associated with a more chronic condition—dementia. It is term used to describe cluster of symptoms, including memory loss (short-and long-term memory), reasoning, judgment, language and other thinking skills. Dementia typically begins slowly, worsens over time and damages a person's abilities in work, social interactions and relationships. When this memory loss disrupts your life, it is one of the first or more-recognizable signs of dementia that may include: repeatedly asking same questions, mixing up words—saying "stove" instead of "refrigerator. Alzheimer's disease is the most common cause of dementia. Alzheimer's disease is characterized by a progressive loss of brain cells and other irregularities of the brain.

Cognitive Decline in the United States

More than 16 million people in the United States are living with cognitive impairment. Researchers found that at least 12% memory loss associated with individuals with depression. Americans 65 and older, about 20 to 25 percent have mild cognitive impairment while about 10 percent have dementia. There are an estimated 5.2 million Americans living with Alzheimer's and research shows that twice as many may be living with the disease but showing no symptoms. Alzheimer's is the third leading cause of death among seniors and is the only disease in the top 10 causes of death with no treatment or cure.

Links to Cognitive Decline

While age is the primary risk factor for cognitive decline, other risk factors include Alzheimer's, brain injury, exposure to pesticides or toxins, physical inactivity, emotional disorders such as depression, anxiety, and stress and chronic conditions such as Parkinson's disease, heart disease and stroke, diabetes, hypothyroidism.

Food Biology of Cognitive Decline (Memory Loss)

When we examine food's role in cognitive decline, we are taking a look at how these foods affect the brain. We learned earlier, there are certain *deficiencies* in neurotransmitters (acetylcholine and dopamine), and nutrients (essential fatty acids, complex carbohydrates, zinc, and probiotic) that have been linked memory loss.

Acetylcholine, the neurotransmitter essential for processing memory and learning, is reduced in both concentration and function in patients with Alzheimer's disease and vascular dementia. Diets high in sugar and saturated fats can suppress dopamine. However, L-tyrosine, an amino acid that helps to build dopamine in the body is a beneficial building block. Zinc plays a pivotal role in communication between neurons in the hippocampus, the brain's learning and memory center. Therefore, zinc mineral deficiency has been linked to cognitive decline. When we experience high levels, or prolonged stress, the stress hormone cortisol is released that cause learning impairments by damaging the cells in the hippocampus which then leads to lowered cognitive functionality and memory loss. A deficiency in essential fatty acids have been linked to memory deficits, especially among individuals with Alzheimer's. It has also been linked to attention deficits, depression, schizophrenia, and Parkinson's disease.

Treatment:

If you're concerned about memory loss, there are tests to determine the degree of memory impairment and diagnose the cause. Problems cognitive decline can be assessed and diagnosed by medical and mental health professionals.

The following are current treatments for cognitive decline:

- **Cognitive behavior therapy (CBT)** can sometimes be effective in teaching strategies to help with managing the effects of impaired function and the diminished capacity that goes with it, in the case of degenerative neurological disorders, such as Alzheimer's or Parkinson's disease it has not shown to be most effective. However, CBT is effective for emotional disorders that causing poor memory.

- **Family support and education** teaches family members about cognitive decline, coping, communication and problem-solving skills. Family members who are informed and involved are more prepared to help loved ones through the process of changes. This is commonly used for Alzheimer's and dementia patients.

- **Medications** control the activity of the neurotransmitter glutamate to improve memory and learning. This is used for individuals with degenerative neurological disorders, such as Alzheimer's.

Optimal Nutritional Suggestions:

As with any treatment, nutrition plays a vital role in our mental well-being. We learned earlier, there are certain deficiencies in neurotransmitters (acetylcholine and dopamine), and nutrients (essential fatty acids, complex carbohydrates, L-tyrosine amino acid, and probiotic) that have been linked to memory loss. It best to avoid sugary drinks, fried foods, processed foods, and alcohol. Let's take a look at food and herbs that contain the protective properties of nutrients that can help with memory loss.

Herbs

- Rosemary
- Ashwagandha
- Gingko Biloba (Maidenhair)
- Periwinkle
- Peppermint
- Ginseng
- Gotu Kola (Indian Pennywort)
- Sage
- Green Tea
- Turmeric
- Black seed oil
- Coconut oil

Foods

- Cold water high-fat fish, Wild Alaskan salmon, Sardines, Trout, Mackerel
- Avocado
- Eggs
- Green leafy vegetables, broccoli, kale, spinach, purslane, mustard greens
- Fiber-rich fruits (apples, strawberries, blueberries, raspberries and bananas)
- Cilantro
- Carrots
- Pineapple
- Acai
- Oranges
- Dark Chocolate
- Plums
- Coconut
- Legumes (lentils, kidney beans, chick peas, split peas, soy beans, pinto beans)

- Fiber-rich grains (buckwheat, wild rice, barley, sorghum, quinoa)
- Nuts (walnuts and brazil nuts)
- Omega-3 EFA oil (Flaxseed or hempseed)
- Seeds (chia, hemp, pumpkin, and sesame)

Water

The recommended water intake is 3.7 liters (15 cups) for the average adult male and 2.7 liters (11 cups) for the average adult female. As discussed previously, the consumption caffeine, sugary drinks, and alcohol causes dehydration which, literally puts a squeeze on the brain. Drinking plenty of water to avoid dehydration also helps to keep cortisol levels lower. Make sure it's purified, alkaline, or spring water.

Mind, Body & Earth Suggestions:

- Of course, exercise is on the list for memory loss. Here's a few ideas exercise:
    - Low-impact: Walking, Yoga, Pilates

- Sleep has a role in the consolidation of memory, which is essential for learning new information. So, make sure you are getting rest! This is beneficial for all mental health problems.

- Here are a few natural crystals with healing properties to help concentration and memory: Carnelian, Black Tourmaline, Citrine, Emerald, Topaz, Aragonite, Snowflake Obsidian, and Fluorite.

MACKEREL PATTIE WITH SPINACH

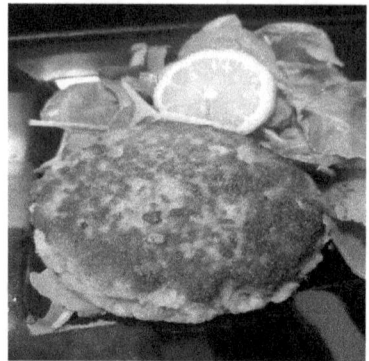

This simple treat is what you need to get your day started with focus. It is great for breakfast or snack.

Ingredients (Serves 4)

- 1 of pound fresh mackerel, skin removed
- ½ cup lemon juice
- 1 $^{1/3}$ cups plain breadcrumbs (Substitute: dry oatmeal)
- 1/3 cup spelt flour
- 1/2 green bell pepper, finely chopped
- 1/2 small onion, finely chopped
- 1/4 cup fresh parsley, chopped
- 1/4 teaspoon sea salt
- 1/8 teaspoon cayenne pepper
- 2 large eggs, lightly beaten
- Coconut Oil

Instructions

1. In a small saucepan, bring 2 cups water and lemon juice to a boil. Add mackerel, cover, and reduce heat to low. Cook for 10 minutes or until salmon is opaque and flaky. Remove salmon and allow to cool.

2. Preheat the oven to 400°F. Line a baking sheet with aluminum foil; set aside.
3. In a large bowl, mix breadcrumbs (oatmeal), spelt flour, bell pepper, onion, parsley, salt, and cayenne.
4. Break apart the mackerel and add to breadcrumb (oatmeal) mixture. Add the egg and mix to combine.
5. Roll a handful of the mixture into a ball and flatten to form a disc.
6. Pray each patty lightly with cooking spray. Place on the prepared baking sheet. Bake for 15 minutes, flipping each patty over halfway through the cooking time. Serve with spinach, asparagus, any leafy green vegetable, or a *Blueberry Boom* salad that you and your family might enjoy!

BLUEBERRY BLOOM SALAD

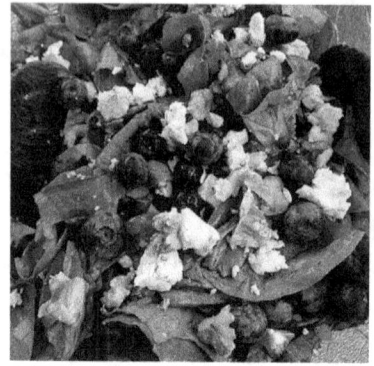

We love salads! As a matter of fact, if you ask co-author, LeAndra, she would say, "Peavy make the best salads!" So, here is recipe for what we call the *Blueberry Boom* because it's packed with antioxidants and omega-3 fatty acids—everything.

Ingredients for Salad (Serves 4)

- 1 bunch of kale, chopped
- 1 bunch of spinach
- 4 oz of cheese crumbles (feta, goat, or blue cheese)
- 1 pint of blueberries
- ½ cup of walnuts
- 1 teaspoon of olive oil

Ingredients for Dressing (Serves 4)

- 1 cup of organic apple cider vinegar (ACV)
- 1 tablespoon of oil (Grapeseed, Hempseed, or Olive)
- ¼ cup of agave nectar
- ½ cup of fresh strawberries (optional)

Instructions

1. Start by cleaning fruit and vegetables in vinegar solution. After chopping kale, toss in 1 tsp of olive oil to soften leaves.

2. Toss in kale, spinach, cheese crumbles, blueberries and walnuts in salad bowl. Chill salad in refrigerator while making dressing.
3. Mix ACV, oil, and agave nectar in glass container. (Optional: Blend strawberries and add to mix).
4. It's time to enjoy your salad!

Chapter 7

Psychosis

"You have to fight in your brain — to argue that what you're believing instinctively is wrong."
~ The Mighty

Understanding Psychosis

Psychosis is a broad term used to describe a mental illness in which the person is experiencing loss of some contact with reality, causing a severe disturbance in thinking, emotion, and behavior. Psychosis can severely impair a person's work, relationships, and ability to function in day-to-day activities, especially self-care. People usually experience psychosis in a myriad of episodic phases which vary in length, it includes premorbid manifestations (no symptoms but at-risk), prodromal (changes that signifies becoming unwell), acute (actively psychotic), recovery (attempt to attain wellness), and relapse (additional episodes following recovery).

There are three major symptoms that a person experiences when psychosis is developing. One of those changes are evolves the person's *mood and drive*—experience of depressive mood, irritability, growing suspicious (paranoia), changes in appetite, anxiety, lack of emotional expression, or inappropriate emotional response. The next noted changes are the person's *rationale and awareness*—experience of weird ideas, odd sensory experience such as reduced or heightened of colors, smells, or sounds (hallucinations); difficulty concentrating, and feelings that self or others have been altered in some way. The other major changes are the person's *behavior*—isolating self from others, inability to function in work or social environment and increased poor sleep habits. Signs and symptoms will vary from person to person and may go undiagnosed for year as so during the early stages. With certain disorders, psychosis occurs secondary, sporadically, or only once during the course of a mental crisis (stressful event).

There are several disorders in which psychosis is a feature: schizophrenia, schizoaffective disorder, bipolar disorder (manic episodes), major depression with psychotic episode, and drug-induced psychosis. In this book, will not explore each of these disorders individually but will examine how food effects the psychotic features of these diseases.

Psychosis in the United States

In the United States, approximately 1% of adults in live with schizophrenia. Nearly 3% of adults live with bipolar disorder and 50% of people have their first episode by age 25. Three out of 100 people will experience psychosis at some point in their lives. Each year about 100,000 adolescents and young adults in the United States experience first episode psychosis.

Links to Psychosis

It is believed psychosis is caused by a combination of factors, including genetics, stress, and biochemistry. Biological factors could be genetic predisposition, changes in brain, or dysfunction the neurotransmitters in the brain.

Food Biology of Psychosis

When we examine food's role in psychosis, we are taking a look at how these foods affect the brain. There are certain *excesses* in neurotransmitters (acetylcholine, serotonin, and dopamine), and *deficiencies* in nutrients (essential fatty acids, complex carbohydrates, Vitamin D, B9, and B12) that have been linked psychosis.

If there is an excess of dopamine in certain regions of the brain, it causes over-stimulation and excessive sensory information which disrupts concentration, thinking, one's reality, emotion, and behavior. Excessive serotonin activity has been linked to hallucination; it is also associated with several disturbances found in psychosis such as poor concentration, aggression, unstable mood, poor appetite, sexual drive, sleep disturbance, and disrupted body movement. When there is excessive acetylcholine in the brain, it causes over-stimulation that results in abnormal excitability (e.g. talking or moving quickly, speaking loudly, laughing uncontrollable).

As mentioned throughout the book, complex carbohydrates help regulate blood sugar (insulin) spikes after a meal which is responsible for hyperactivity and poor concentration. Correcting blood sugar problems is paramount in managing psychosis. Therefore, diet must be sufficient in complex carbohydrates—fiber and starch. Research found that individuals with psychosis have low level of essential fatty acids (EFAs). A deficiency of B12 has been linked to hallucinations, irritability, paranoia, and thought fogginess including memory loss. A deficiency in essential fatty acids have been linked to schizophrenia as well as inattentiveness, depressive mood, and neurological disorders such as

Alzheimer's disease and Parkinson's disease. As stated throughout this book, simple carbohydrates such as raw sugar, brown sugar, corn syrup and high-fructose corn syrup, glucose, fructose, and sucrose, or fruit juice concentrate should be avoided as in will likely increase psychotic symptoms.

Treatment:

Psychosis can be assessed and diagnosed by medical and mental health professionals. Psychosis is best treated by a team of professionals. The course and length of treatment will be slightly different for someone with a brief psychotic episode rather someone who experiences psychosis chronically. The following are current treatments for psychosis:

The following are current treatments for Psychosis:

- **Antipsychotic medications** help reduce psychosis symptoms. Like all medications, antipsychotic drugs have risks and benefits. The treating psychiatrists can discuss side effects and dosage preferences such as taking daily pills or monthly injection.

- **Psychotherapy or Cognitive behavior therapy (CBT)** help clients identify the defenses they utilize against intolerable feelings of loss or failure; identify distorted or unhelpful thinking patterns, recognize and change inaccurate beliefs, relate to others in more positive ways, and change problematic behaviors, respectively.

➤ **Family support and education** teaches family members about psychosis, coping, communication and problem-solving skills. Family members who are informed and involved are better equipped to help loved ones through the challenging process to recovery.

➤ **Supported Employment/Education (SEE)** services help clients enter the workforce or school and achieve their personal goals. The chief concern is on rapid placement for work or school, combined with coaching and support to success in those placements.

➤ **Case Management** helps clients develop and practice problem-solving. Case managers often offer solutions to address day-to-day problems and organize social services to address client's multiple needs.

Optimal Nutritional Suggestions:

As with any treatment, nutrition plays a vital role in our mental well-being. There are certain excesses in acetylcholine, serotonin, dopamine and deficiencies in essential fatty acids, complex carbohydrates, Vitamin D, B9, and B12 that have been linked psychosis. Diet changes do not always make a difference for people with chronic psychosis because of other factors such as using tobacco. Let's take a look at food and herbs that contain the protective properties of nutrients that can help elevate distressing symptoms psychosis.

Herbs
- Dandelion
- Sage

- Gingko Biloba (Maidenhair)
- Damiana

Foods

- Cold water high-fat fish (wild Alaskan salmon, sardines, anchovies, mackerel, shad, herring, and trout)
- Turkey and Chicken (dark meat)
- Shellfish (shrimp, lobster, oysters, crab)
- Avocado
- Alfalfa
- Dark green leafy vegetables (kale, spinach, purslane, mustard greens, and collards)
- Fiber-rich fruits (apples, strawberries, blueberries, raspberries and bananas)
- Melons
- Lemon
- Mushrooms
- Milk
- Eggs
- Beans (lentils, kidney beans, chick peas, split peas, soy beans, pinto beans)
- Fiber-rich grains (buckwheat, wild rice, barley, sorghum, quinoa)
- Nuts (walnuts and brazil nuts)
- Omega-3 EFA oil (Flaxseed or hempseed)
- Seeds (hempseeds, pumpkin, and sesame)

Mind, Body & Earth Suggestions:

➢ Exercise produce endorphins (chemicals in the brain that act as natural painkillers). It doesn't matter what type of physical activity as long as you get moving for at least 30 minutes for three to five days per week. Here's a few ideas for any fitness level:

- Low-Impact: Walking, Yoga, Jogging, Cycling

➢ Deep Breathing. This is helpful to manage tension that comes with dealing distressing thoughts.

- See page 69 for instructions on proper technique.

➢ Progressive Muscle Relaxation (PMR).

- (1) Sit back or lie down in a comfortable position. Close your eyes if you're comfortable doing so. (2) Beginning at your feet, notice how your muscles feel. Are they tense, or relaxed? (3) Tightly tense the muscles in your feet by curling your toes. Hold the tension for 5-10 seconds. (4) Release the tension from your feet and allow them to relax. Focus on how different the states of tension and relaxation feel. (5) Move up your body, repeating the cycle of tensing and relaxing each group of muscles. Be sure to practice on the following groups of muscles: legs, pelvis, stomach, chest, back, arms, hands, neck, and face. (6) Practice daily — at any time. PMR is great for combating depression and anxiety, too!

➢ Here are a few natural crystals with healing properties to help concentration and memory: Unakite, Orange Calcite, Tiger's Eye, Smokey Quartz, and Amber.

GREEN BERRY SMOOTHIE

This smoothie is filled with antioxidants, vitamins, and minerals to protect your brain health. It's delicious, too!

Ingredients (Serves 2)

- ½ cup of kale
- 1 cup of spinach
- 1 large banana, peeled
- 2 apples, cored and cut
- 1 ½ cups of strawberries, frozen
- 2 tablespoons flaxseeds, grounded
- 2 cups of purified water
- 1 tablespoon of agave nectar (optional)

Instructions

1. Start by cleaning berries of pesticides. Fill a large bowl with 4 parts water to 1 part plain white vinegar. Soak the berries in the mixture for 20 minutes. Then rise.
2. Place kale, spinach, and water into blender. Blend until you have green juice consistency.
3. Stop blending and add your other ingredients. Blend until you have a creamy smoothie. Give a taste for desired sweetness. If the apples and banana did not sweeten enough, add your sweetener. (NO sugar, please.)
4. Enjoy your delicious smoothie!

GROUND TURKEY SLAM

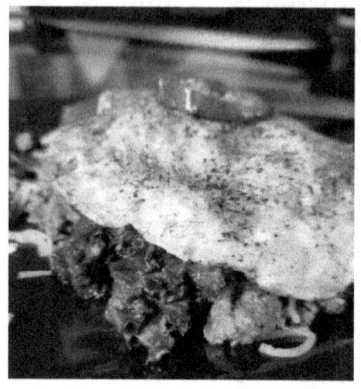

This is Dr. Peavy's favorite brunch delight. It is packed with nutrients you need to protect your brain. Turkey has the amino acid, tryptophan, and kale has fiber, calcium, and vitamin C to help boost antioxidant levels to protect brain.

Ingredients (Serves 4)

- 4 Organic Free-Range Egg (Alternative: Egg White)
- 1 pound of organic ground turkey
- 1 bunch of cleaned and chopped kale
- 1 teaspoon minced garlic powder
- 1 chopped onion
- 1 teaspoon of sage
- 1 teaspoon of cracked black pepper
- 1 teaspoon of sea salt (optional)
- 1 tablespoon of grapeseed oil (omega-6)
- 1 cup of low-fat shredded cheese (optional)
- Jalapeno (optional)

Instructions

1. Season thawed ground turkey with garlic, sage, pepper and sea salt (optional).

2. Heat oil in a large skillet over medium-high heat. Add diced onions and cook until soft. Crumble ground turkey and garlic into the pan and cook until turkey is browned.
3. Heat oil in pan over low-medium heat. Add kale and season to your taste. Sauté to your desired texture (but don't overcook).
4. Heat dash of oil in small skillet for fried eggs. Season and fry each egg separately to your desire. Le'Andra enjoys her egg over-easy and Dr. Peavy sunny side up.
5. Place a serving of ground turkey on the plate, top with shredded cheese (optional), top with kale, and a fried egg. You may garnish with a slice of jalapeno for spice (optional).
6. Enjoy this goodness!

REFERENCES

American Psychiatric Association. Diagnostic and Statistical Manual of Mental Disorders, Fifth Edition. Arlington, VA: American Psychiatric Publishing, 2013 [accessed 2018 AUG 21].

American Psychiatric Association. Practice Guidelines for the Treatment of Patients With Major Depressive Disorder, Third Edition. Arlington, VA: American Psychiatric Publishing, 2010 [accessed 2018 AUG 21].

Anglin, R., Samaan, Z., Walter, S., & McDonald, S. (2013). Vitamin D deficiency and depression in adult: Systematic review and meta-analysis. The British Journal of Psychiatry, 202, 100-107.

Bear T, Philipp M, Hill S, Mündel T. A preliminary study on how hypohydration affects pain perception. Psychophysiology. 2016 May; 53(5):605-10.

Berry N, Robinson M, Bryan J, Buckley J, Murphy K, Howe P. (2011). Acute effects of an Avena sativa herb extract on responses to the Stroop Color-Word test. J Altern Complement Med. Jul; 17(7):635-7.

Bourre, J (2006). Effects of nutrients (in food) on the structure and function of the nervous system: update on dietary requirements for brain: Part 1: micronutrients. J. Nutrition, Health & Aging: Vol 10(5), 377-385.

Center for Behavioral Health Statistics and Quality. (2015). Behavioral health trends in the United States: Results from the 2014 National Survey on Drug Use and Health (HHS Publication No. SMA 15-4927, NSDUH Series H-50).

Coppen, A (2000). .Enhancement of antidepressant action of fluoxetine by folic acid: a randomized, placebo controlled trial. J Affect Disord. (60), 121-130.

Davidson, M., Caspi, A., & Noy, S. (2005). The treatment of schizophrenia: from premorbid manifestations to the first episode of psychosis. Dialogues in clinical neuroscience, 7(1), 7-16.

Di Pasquale MG. The essentials of essential fatty acids. J Diet Suppl. 2009;6(2):143-61.

Foster JA, McVey Neufeld KA. (2013). Gut-brain axis: how the microbiome influences anxiety and depression. Trends Neurosci. May; 36(5):305-12.

Gonzalez-Estecha M, Trasobares EM, Tajima K, et al. (2011). Trace elements in bipolar disorder. *J. Trace. Elem. Med. Biol* 25 Suppl 1, S78-83.

Harris, S. (2016, April). Vitamin D and African-Americans. The Journal of Nutrition, 136 (4), 1126-1129.

Hedelin, M. (2010). Dietary Intake of Fish, Omega 3's, Omega 6 PUFA's and Vitamin D and the Prevalence of Psychotic Symptoms in a Cohort of 33,000 Women from the General Population. BMC Psychiatry (10): 38; 1-13

Hubbarda, NA, Hutchisonab, JL, Turnera, M, Montroyc, J, Bowlesc RP, and Rypmaab, V. (2015). Depressive thoughts limit working memory capacity in dysphoria. Journal of Cognition & Emotion.

Judd et al. (2003).Long-term symptomatic status of bipolar I vs II disorders. Int J Neuropsychopharm. 6(2):127-37.

Li Y, et. al (2017). Dietary patterns and depression risk: A meta-analysis. *Psychiatry Res.* Jul; 253:373-382

MacQueen GM, Memedovich KA. (2017). Cognitive dysfunction in major depression and bipolar disorder, Assessment and treatment options. Psychiatry. *Clin. Neurosci* 71, 18-27.

Maes M.Et.al. (1999). Lower serum zinc in major depression in relation to changes in serum acute phase proteins. *J. Affect Disord.* 56(2-3):189-194.

Oades, Robert. (2010). *The Role of Serotonin in Attention-Deficit Hyperactivity Disorder (ADHD)*. Handbook of Behavioral Neuroscience. 21. 565-584.

Quehl R, Haines J, Lewis SP, Buchholz AC. (2017). Food and mood: diet quality is inversely associated with depressive symptoms in female university students. Can J Diet Pract ;78:124–8.

Raupp, A.E. (2018). Body Belief: How to Heal Autoimmune Diseases, Radically Shift Your Health, and Learn to Love Your Body More. Hay House: New York.

Wilkins CH., et al.: (2006). Vitamin D deficiency is associated with low mood and worse cognitive performance in older adults. *Am J Geriatric Psychiatry*, Dec; 14(12):1032-1040

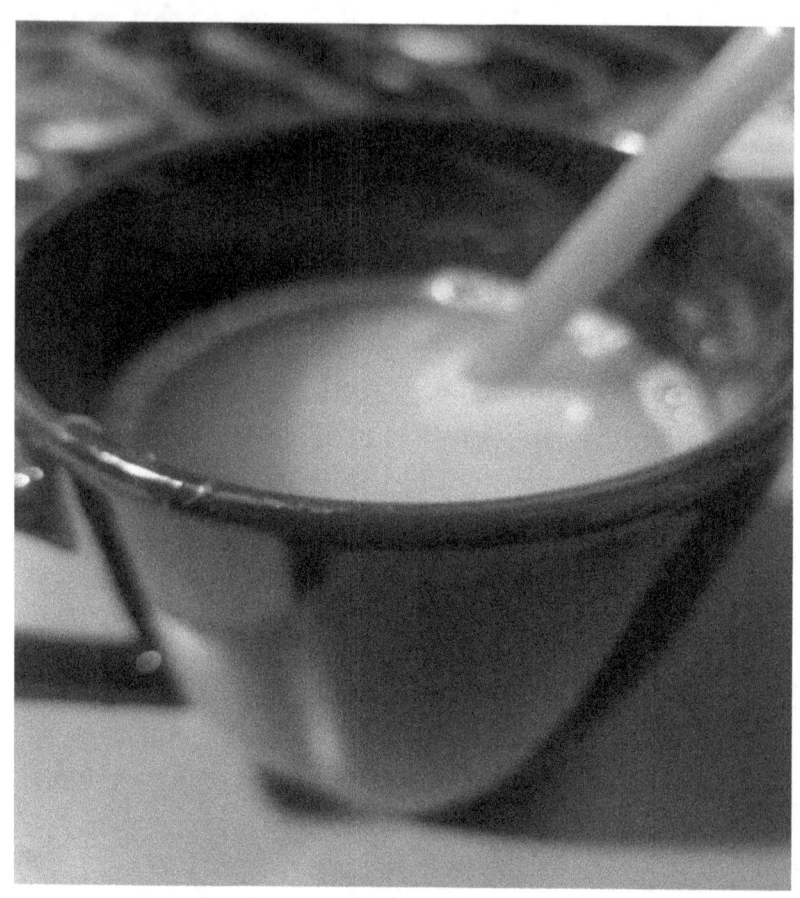

The TEA!

Here is a list of herbs that are used to make tea to assist with anxiety, depression and even, sleep! We did not include a chapter specifically for sleep because many times poor sleep is a symptom of other behavioral health concerns we covered in this book. Therefore, sleep disturbances should improve with new dietary changes. Sip tea and live well!

Herbs

- Blue Vervain (stress, depression and restlessness.)
- Prodigiosa (anxiety)
- Bugleweed (anxiety)
- Valerian (anxiety, nervousness, exhaustion and hysteria)
- Linden (depression and insomnia)
- Damiana (anxiety, nervousness, and depression)
- Lavendar (anxiety and insomnia)
- Turmeric (depression, anxiety, brain fog, ADHD, and memory loss, as well as neurological diseases such as Alzheimer's).

Ingredients (Servings 2)

- Choose your desired herb.
- 2 cups of purified water
- 1 teaspoon of agave nectar (optional)
- 1 lemon (optional)

Instructions for loose leaves

1. Choose herb.
2. Boil in water for 20 minutes.
3. Place 4 tsp. of herbal buds into a tea ball (or sachet).
4. Place the tea ball and water into a teacup.
5. Strain and serve.

Instructions for herbal powder

1. Choose herbal powder.
2. Heat in water for 5 minutes.
3. Place herbal powder into mug and add water.
5. Add lemon, and/or sweetener.

You can maintain your body and brain health by making healthy choices about your lifestyle—diet, exercise and self-care. The choice you make can help prevent and minimize the impact of disease.

Thank you for taking stock in this guide, but most importantly—taking stock in yourself and your tribe.

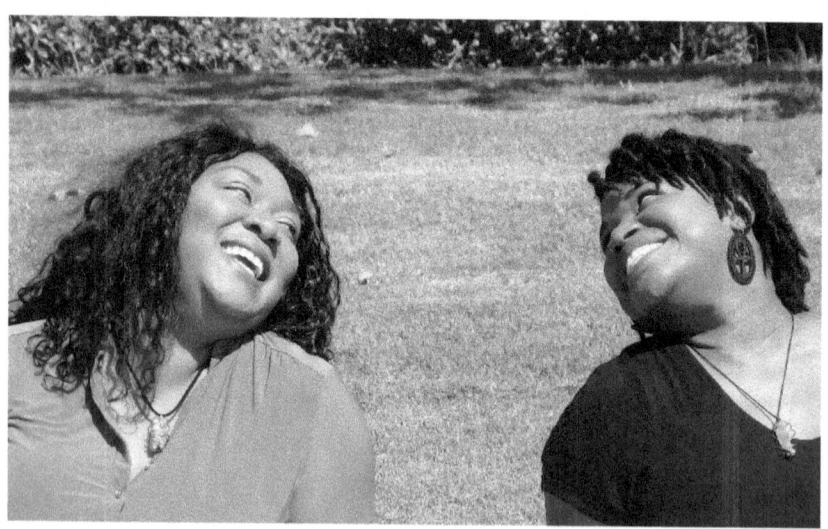

JOURNAL

Keep track of food and herbs that you've food beneficial.

Food/Herb	Notes

Mental Health Resources

General Mental Health Resources
- Mental Health America: www.mentalhealthamerica.net
  Free mental screenings and other resources
- Therapy for Black Girls: www.therapyforblackgirls.com
- Psychology Today: www.psychologytoday.com
  - Nationwide listings for mental health professionals

Depression
- National Suicide Prevention Lifeline: 1-800-273-TALK (8255)
  - Hearing impaired: 1-800-799-4889
- National Youth Crisis Hotline: 1-800-448-4663

Stress & Anxiety
- National Center for PTSD: www.ptsd.va.gov
- The Calm Clinic: www.calmclinic.com

Cognitive Decline (Memory Loss)
- Alzheimer's Association: www.alz.org

Veteran Mental Health
- The Boris Lawrence Henson Foundation: www.borislhensonfoundation.org

Note: We are not responsible for the content, claims or representations of the listed sites.